More praise for

Strong Women and Men *Beat Arthritis*

"As an athlete who has had injuries, I am concerned about my muscles and joints. This is a program that is easy to follow. *Strong Women and Men Beat Arthritis* provides the tools and motivation to keep my joints healthy as I grow older." —Pam Shriver, tennis champion

"This clearly written self-care manual by Nelson . . . and her colleagues . . . should be a boon to arthritis sufferers . . . Extremely helpful."

—*Publishers Weekly*

"Clear, practica[...] [...] take control of their arthrit[...] [...] Klippel, M.D., [...]tis Foundation

"Scientifically [...] [...]o follow, and clearly written. [...]

[...]senberg, M.D., Dea[...] [...]fts University

"Provides com[...] [...]n shows you how to do it—[...] [...]rence Lindner, [...]utrition Letter

"Up-to-date s[...] [...]excellent resource to help [...] [...]th, regardless of their age." [...] C. Raymond, [...]is Foundation

"I will strongly [...] [...]cerned about their bones—it [...] [...]actical."
—Robert Neer, M.D., director, Osteoporosis Center, Massachusetts General Hospital

"Nelson's powerful upbeat message will get even couch potatoes on their feet and pumping iron." —*Time*

continued on next page . . .

Strong Women Stay Young

"An essential tool for women of all ages." —C. Everett Koop, M.D., former United States Surgeon General

"A vitally important book, based on solid scientific research, which for the first time offers hope to the woman who wants to live a long, vigorously active and healthy life to the fullest. It shows clearly that many of the changes associated with aging can be not only delayed, but even reversed."

—Kenneth H. Cooper, M.D., MPH, author of *The Aerobics Program for Total Well-Being*

"Dr. Nelson has provided women an outstanding opportunity to grow stronger, healthier, and younger." —William J. Evans, Ph.D., director, Nutrition, Metabolism, and Exercise Laboratory at the University of Arkansas for Medical Sciences, and author of *Biomarkers*

"A terrific book! Finally, a science-based program to help women of all ages live strong and vital lives." —Robert N. Butler, M.D., director, International Longevity Center, Mount Sinai Medical Center

Strong Women Stay Slim

"This book is a gem . . . thoroughly based in science, yet written to help women get started immediately to make their lives better today. It's jam-packed with ready-to-go tools for success."

—Barbara Harris, editor in chief, *Shape* magazine

"This book is a winner! Miriam Nelson shows women how to take charge and lose weight from a position of strength. Finally there's a weight-loss program that appeals to our intelligence and promotes our fitness."

—Billie Jean King, tennis champion

ALSO BY MIRIAM E. NELSON, PH.D.
(WITH SARAH WERNICK, PH.D.)

Strong Women Stay Young

Strong Women Stay Slim

Strong Women, Strong Bones

(WITH JUDY KNIPE)

Strong Women Eat Well

MIRIAM E. NELSON, PH.D.,

KRISTIN R. BAKER, PH.D., AND

RONENN ROUBENOFF, M.D., M.H.S.,

with

LAWRENCE LINDNER, M.A.

A PERIGEE BOOK

Strong Women

and Men

Beat Arthritis

◆

THE SCIENTIFICALLY PROVEN PROGRAM THAT ALLOWS PEOPLE WITH ARTHRITIS TO TAKE CHARGE OF THEIR DISEASE

Sources for the nutrient data in the book are from the USDA Nutrient Database (http://www.nal.usda.gov/fnic/) and from the program "Diet Analysis Plus" by West/Wadsworth Publishing Company and ESHA Research.

X-rays on pages 14–15 reprinted with permission from D. M. Forrester, M.D., and J. C. Brown, M.D., *The Radiology of Joint Disease* (Philadelphia: W. B. Saunders Company, 1987).

PAR-Q questionnaire on pages 90–91 reprinted with permission of Canadian Society for Exercise Physiology.

Exercise intensity scales on pages 96 and 150 used with permission from Miriam E. Nelson, Ph.D., with Sarah Wernick, Ph.D., *Strong Women Stay Young* (New York: Bantam Books, 2000).

Readiness questionnaire on page 173 adapted with permission from Bess Marcus et al., *Health Psychology* 1992; 11(6):386–95.

Sources for costs of medications from Tarascon ePharmacopoeia and from local pharmacies.

A Perigee Book
Published by The Berkley Publishing Group
A division of Penguin Putnam Inc.
375 Hudson Street
New York, New York 10014

G. P. Putnam's Sons edition: April 2002
First Perigee edition: March 2003

Perigee trade paperback edition ISBN: 0-399-52856-3

Visit our website at www.penguinputnam.com

The Library of Congress has catalogued the
G. P. Putnam's Sons hardcover edition as follows:

Nelson, Miriam E.
Strong women and men beat arthritis / Miriam E. Nelson, Kristin R. Baker,
and Ronenn Roubenoff, with Lawrence Lindner.
p. cm.
Includes bibliographical references and index.
ISBN 0-399-14852-3
1. Arthritis—Popular works. I. Baker, Kristin R., date. II. Roubenoff, Ronenn. III. Title.

RC993.N455   2002   2001048487
616.7'22—dc21

Printed in the United States of America

10 9 8 7 6 5 4 3 2

*We dedicate this book to Liz, Sister Mary Patrice, Deborah,
and all of the other study volunteers who have given so much
in the hope that the research will help others with arthritis.*

An Important Caution

■

The "Strong Women *and Men* Beat Arthritis" program is based on extensive scientific research. This book contains instructions and safety precautions. It is essential that you read them carefully. Some exercises are inappropriate for individuals with severe arthritis or other medical conditions.

This book is not intended to replace the services of a health-care provider who knows you personally. An essential element of taking responsibility for your health is having regular checkups and working in partnership with medical professionals.

If you are under treatment for arthritis or any other medical condition—or if you suspect you might need such care—you must discuss this program with your doctor before you begin.

Contents

■

Acknowledgments

■

A ll books are a team effort, no matter how few names appear on the cover. This book is no exception. First, we are indebted to the dean of the Gerald J. and Dorothy R. Friedman School of Nutrition Science and Policy at Tufts University, Dr. Irwin Rosenberg, for his continued support of our research as well as our efforts to get our results out into the public domain so that people can make the best use of them.

Numerous other colleagues at Tufts have also been enormously helpful. We single out Dr. Laura Rall, Joe Walsmith, Jennifer Layne, Leslie Abad, and Nancy Lungren for their research expertise and Felina Mucha-Cyr for her willingness in taking on administrative and other responsibilities necessary for the successful completion of this book. To Rebecca Seguin, we express particular gratitude for her aid in gathering resources, tying up loose ends (especially at the end!), and vetting and editing various portions of the manuscript.

Many thanks go to the scientists and physicians at the Perlman Family Arthritis Center at the New England Medical Center who over the years have always been willing to help in more ways than can be mentioned: Allen Steere, M.D.; Elena Massarotti, M.D.; Nathalie Boileau, M.D.; Samantha Cunha, R.N.; Bernadette Muldoon, R.N.; and Paul Dellaripa, M.D.

A special thank-you to David Felson, M.D., M.P.H., of the National Institutes of Health Multipurpose Arthritis and Musculoskeletal Diseases Center at Boston University Medical School. David was an invaluable collaborator on our exercise study targeting people with osteoarthritis, and he continues to direct Kristin's research efforts.

Gracious thanks go to the Charles H. Farnsworth Trust at the Medical Foundation, the Arthritis Foundation, the American Federation of Aging Research Glenn Foundation, N.I.H., U.S.D.A., and Life Fitness for their generous support of the research that forms the basis of this book.

Our colleagues at Putnam also have been incredibly supportive. Stacy Creamer and Jennifer Repo, our editors, offered keen insight and helped keep us on track throughout the process. Marilyn Ducksworth and the others in the publicity department at Putnam have unfailingly kept the *Strong Women* books in the news, helping to get our message out there.

Wendy Weil, our fantastic agent, has been an ardent supporter—and great friend—right from the start. And Wendy Wray's wonderful illustrations once again grace the *Strong Women* pages. Her talent is no small part of our ability to get our exercises across to the reader in the clearest manner possible. Neill Walsdorf, Jr., and his colleagues at Mission Pharmacal have been enthusiastic supporters of Miriam's work and helped to promote the *Strong Women* mission worldwide. Kevin Bart, Miriam's public-relations director, has tirelessly and creatively kept Miriam and *Strong Women* in the public eye.

Colleagues at the *Tufts University Health & Nutrition Letter,* both past and present, are more appreciated than they know for their encouragement and their "ear." They include (but are not limited to) Gail Zyla, whose friendship is worth more than words; Deborah White, whose trust has always allowed for the necessary creativity; and Anne Fletcher, who never hesitated to instill confidence and who taught us early on that what goes around comes around—especially the good things! A special thanks here to Christine Smith, whose patience, flexibility, and goodwill were crucial to the writing of this book.

Numerous individuals agreed to be interviewed for this work, passing on their stories so that other people with arthritis could be motivated to receive the benefits of our program. A thousand thank-yous, in particular, to Liz, Sister Mary Patrice, Deborah, Earl, Fred, and Mark.

To Heather, Joe, David, Judy, and Arlene go much appreciation for serving as wonderful models for our illustrator. Your work is no small part of this endeavor.

We thank here, too, a number of behind-the-scenes people who were instrumental in planting the seeds for this book: Sally Nelson, Bill and Lisa Nelson, Carly and Warren Baker, Dbora Roubenoff and the late Robert Roubenoff, and Shirley and Raymond Lindner.

Of course, thanks stronger than we could adequately express go to our incredibly patient and supportive spouses: Kin Earle, Corey Peck, Abby Shevitz, and Constance Lindner. Without you, this book simply would not have been written.

Finally, our children deserve special acknowledgment for putting up with our absences during the long writing process. Thanks, Mason, Eliza, Alexandra, Ethan, McKenna, and little John Matthew, who accommodated us enormously by synchronizing his gestation with the gestation of this book.

Preface

∎

Only a few times in a scientist's career can he or she expect the results of a study to be much more successful than originally hypothesized. That is exactly what happened in the study that forms the foundation for this book.

Several years ago I received funding to investigate the effects of strength training for relieving the pain of arthritis. To help me conduct this study, I turned to my lab chief and close friend, Dr. Ronenn Roubenoff. Ronenn is a board-certified rheumatologist with more than a decade of experience working with arthritis patients—as well as a phenomenal scientist. I also turned to my talented doctoral fellow, Kristin Baker, who had worked in our laboratory for several years and had a keen interest in arthritis. The three of us, along with other collaborators, designed and conducted the study. As you will see when you read the book, the program we designed made a tremendous difference in the lives of arthritis sufferers.

Once the results were published, I felt strongly that I wanted to get the program out to the widest possible audience. So I decided to write this book. Working together with Ronenn and Kristin and drawing on the writing expertise of another colleague at Tufts, Larry Lindner, we put this book together so that arthritis sufferers could benefit from the latest research not only in exercise but also in nutrition, medical management, surgery, and complementary therapies.

Kristin, Ronenn, and I have all seen firsthand what a difference changes in lifestyle can make for individuals with arthritis. For us, this book is a chance to make a difference outside the academic ivory tower in a way that a hundred scientific articles never could.

SECTION I

New Strategies for Dealing with Arthritis

CHAPTER 1

You Can Reduce the Pain

■

Even to roll over, the pain woke me up. I was so depressed. I had just re-signed myself to the fact that I couldn't do much. My doctor had written in his notes, "Liz is depressed, debilitated." When I saw that, it really made me want to cry.

—LIZ, 46

My left knee had been hurting since my late fifties. Nothing seemed to work. By 10:00 in the morning, I had pain in my leg. I could never take a walk without stopping. It was hard to drive. My knee would stiffen.

—SISTER MARY PATRICE, 71

My hip felt like it was burning, combined with a dull ache. I was think-ing about the pain all the time, resigned to the fact that I had a pretty shabby quality of life ahead of me.

—FRED, 37

FORTY-THREE MILLION PEOPLE HAVE ARTHRITIS

Whether you have arthritis yourself or know someone else who has it, you are intimately familiar with the pain it can inflict, the depression, and sometimes the sense of hopelessness. You're by no means alone: Nearly everyone knows at least a couple of people with arthritis. Forty-three million Americans are afflicted with the disease, which results in as much disability as conditions like heart disease, diabetes, and hip fractures. Indeed, fully half of those affected are disabled within 10 years, while one in fourteen is hospitalized.

It's a constant struggle. Arthritis, along with back pain, is the number-two reason people see their doctors, after colds and flus, and in older adults it causes more difficulty with day-to-day activities—such as walking—than any other disease. These are no small details. And the prevalence of arthritis increases with age: Nearly half of adults over age 65 have it.

Unfortunately, there are a couple of myths about arthritis that get in the way of treatment—treatment that can reduce pain and even give people their lives back.

Myth: Rest is best.

This myth comes from some circles in the medical community itself. There are still a lot of doctors who believe that rest is the best treatment for the disease. It's not. But unfortunately the misinformation gets handed from doctor to patient. In one study conducted at the Harvard School of Public Health, researchers reported that in only half of the encounters between patients with rheumatoid arthritis and their rheumatologists was exercise even discussed. And in a study in Canada, where family physicians see most arthritis patients, only a third of the doctors queried recommended exercise to people with arthritis of the knee.

Granted, some research studies do show that certain types of exercises can contribute to the development of arthritis. But that's in elite athletes who push their bodies to the brink.

Research from our own laboratory at Tufts University as well as from other scientific institutions makes it quite clear that the *right* types of exercise, performed correctly, actually restore people's function while dramatically cutting down on their pain.

Myth: My joints are too far gone to make a difference.

Another myth that prevents people with arthritis from getting help circulates among many sufferers themselves. Patients often ask themselves, "What can I expect at this stage of the game?"

Our answer: Plenty! In fact, not just young adults in pain but also people in their sixties, seventies, and older can absolutely turn their lives around by taking the proper steps to shore up arthritic joints. But don't take our word for it. Listen to the comments of the arthritis sufferers quoted above, who eventually followed our program:

■ ■ ■

I remember the days when I'd think, How I am I going to maneuver myself out of the bed? *Now it's just,* Get up and go. *It's unbelievable. My whole outlook is different. Before, I couldn't get up to answer the phone, but just yesterday, I got out of the car and ran across the road to get the mail. My sister said, "I haven't seen you run in years." I keep being able to do more and more. Even the mood in the house is lighter. We're able to do more things as a family.*

—LIZ

My energy level became so much better. It just made such a big difference. I had no pain medication at all. It's such a wonderful feeling, being able to walk up and down the stairs—right foot, left foot, instead of just one foot. The walking is so much better. People notice the difference. My energy level is great, too. I can feel the strength in my legs.

—SISTER MARY PATRICE

I noticed an effect in about three weeks—pretty fast. I've been able to go from not doing any exercise at all to exercising on an elliptical trainer or stationary bike. It's a quite dramatic reduction in pain—almost like you don't think about it anymore. I can even get more work done.

—FRED

■ ■ ■

THE SCIENTIFIC PROGRAM THAT WILL GIVE YOU YOUR LIFE BACK

What is it, exactly, that can so turn people's lives around, freeing them from the physical disability and depression that all too often accompany arthritis?

Amazingly, it's largely *a series of lifestyle steps that are entirely in your own control.* The cornerstone of those steps is a plan we've developed that includes exercise, nutrition, and, when necessary, medication.

The exercise component

A lot of Americans, as you already know, are very sedentary, and have been for many years—even decades. So the idea of exercise is daunting to them, to say the least. They cannot imagine themselves finding the energy to challenge their bodies or work up a sweat. They think that lifting weights, walking, or engaging in other forms of activity is only for people who are already fit. In their minds, you're either a "jock" or a "couch potato" with very little room in between. Many older people, in particular, are afraid of the rapid breathing that exercise can cause; they see it as dangerous and uncomfortable.

The thinking that exercise would be physically too demanding and overwhelming is probably even more true among people with arthritis, which makes perfect sense. Many are very out of shape, and some are overweight. It hurts just to walk up a flight of stairs or lift groceries out of the car. There's also the self-consciousness that accompanies moving around when you don't feel good about the shape you're in. So it's not at all surprising that the last thing you might feel up to when you are in pain is putting pressure on your body to make it perform better.

But believe us, anticipating all the discomfort of exercise and the adjustment to a more active lifestyle is much, much worse than actually engaging in the change. Think of anything in your life that you were afraid of doing but then finally tried and loved. Maybe it was jumping off a diving board, or participating in a club or other organization, or changing jobs. Just considering it may have been nerve-wracking enough to make you sweat, but once you tried it, you never knew how you lived without the pleasure it brought.

It's the same with our exercise plan. Once you start, you'll feel so much better you'll never want to go back to being sedentary. And it's not just because exercise helps relieve stress on arthritic joints (more on that in Chapter 3). Just look at all the other benefits exercise brings:

Exercise . . .
- tones the body by building muscle (which in turn burns body fat).
- relieves depression. (Did you know that 12 percent of women are clinically depressed, but research studies have proven that exercise improves and sometimes even eliminates depression?)
- increases flexibility.
- improves balance.
- strengthens bone.
- boosts self-confidence and self-esteem, which in turn help you to continue to exercise.

Exercise even restores vitality and vigor, even though many people believe it will sap them of energy. Imagine mitigating arthritis pain as well as enjoying all those other advantages. Most of the people we work with say that taking up an exercise program has made them feel 20 years younger!

The best part: We make incorporating exercise into your lifestyle as easy as it can possibly be, progressing very, very gradually. In fact, every single strength-training exercise we give you starts out with an easy version for people who need to build up their strength and only moves on to more challenging versions when *you* determine that you're ready. You'll be pushed, yes, but not challenged beyond your limit.

All in the comfort of your own home
A number of studies have shown that when people come to a lab or other research facility and follow an exercise program under the guidance of a trained professional, they do very well. But when the program ends, so does the exercise—there's no one there to keep folks' motivation up, and there's no more access to the fancy equipment that all the exercises were performed on.

That's where our program is different. At Tufts we conducted a definitive study which demonstrated that people can exercise to decrease arthritis pain and increase their ability to function right in their own homes. That's right. One of us, Kristin Baker, went to the homes of dozens of people—women and men who all had osteoarthritis—and showed them how to work with very simple, inexpensive equipment that can be purchased in any sporting goods store. We will discuss the study, which was published in the *Journal of Rheumatology,* in more detail in Chapter 3.

What it means is that you won't be *simulating* what our study participants were doing. You'll be doing exactly the same things in your own living room, family room, basement, or bedroom. That's because we'll be recommending the same exercises with the same equipment.

Of course, Kristin won't be able to come to your home and show you how to do each exercise in person. But there is even more detail in this book than we gave our volunteers, so we *know* you can do it. We've even devoted an entire chapter to motivation that you can consult as often as necessary to keep you going. Think of it as a stand-in for Kristin's visits.

The bottom line: You'll have everything you need. You won't have to adapt the program to accommodate your situation at home. The exercise program is *designed* for you at home.

The nutrition component

Research studies have pointed to various foods—as well as specific nutrients—that can ameliorate arthritis pain. But each study stood on its own. No one ever looked at how one fit with another and then translated them into an overall dietary *pattern* for use in everyday menus—until now. We have reviewed the research and put together an overall eating plan that not only will diminish your arthritis symptoms but also will have a positive impact on numerous other aspects of your health, including your risks for heart disease and diabetes. Specifically, in Chapter 4 we've created an Arthritis Food Guide Pyramid that tells you exactly how much to eat every day in the way of grains, fruits and vegetables, and other foods. There'll be no guesswork on your part. We even give sample menu plans so you can see what a day's worth of meals and snacks might look like if you're following, for instance, a 2,000-calorie plan or a 1,600-calorie plan. And we suggest what dietary supplements to try in conjunction with your foods.

Don't worry—we won't be sending you to the health-food store for foods and ingredients that you're not familiar with or that don't taste good. Our recommended diet is easy to construct, with nearly every ingredient available right at your supermarket, and if it's not at your local market, we'll tell you where in your locale you're likely to be able to find it or how to order it.

You might be surprised at how modifying your diet to protect your joints can potentially cut down on stiffness and inflammation. And the changes are not so drastic that you'll have to eat differently from the rest of your family. In fact, anyone in your household can eat this way and will likely end up healthier for it.

By following our diet, you will also have the opportunity to lose any excess pounds you might be carrying—a crucial step since excess weight can add extra stress to joints in the knees and hips, making arthritis all the more uncomfortable.

The medication component

Drugs are tricky substances. On the one hand, better ones are being developed all the time that can target afflicted joints and thereby reduce inflammation, redness, stiffness, and, ultimately, pain. On the other hand, just about all drugs have side effects. And often, the more powerful the drug, the more complicated its "down side." No wonder some people don't take prescribed or recommended drugs, even though they can diminish their arthritis pain. They are afraid of the side effects.

But if you understand exactly which drugs work in what way and how they affect your body—as well as how to head off or lessen side effects—you're in a much better position to work with your health-care provider on controlling pain without introducing new problems. That's why, in Chapter 7, we lay out in clear terms exactly how medications work, their side effects, and how to deal with those effects whenever possible. We even include discussions on the cost of drugs with suggestions for how to decide when a prescription drug might be less expensive than an over-the-counter medication and vice versa.

Of course, while a particular drug can sometimes have a dramatic impact on a person's quality of life, generally speaking, no drug can do everything by itself. We have found that it's most often the *synergy* resulting from a combination of the right exercise program, the right nutrition program, and the right medication(s) that offers the most relief. Taking a drug without exercising and eating properly usually produces only a fraction of the best possible effect.

Complementary therapies

Reducing arthritis pain doesn't necessarily have to stop with exercise, nutrition, and medication. Many people are now trying a variety of complementary therapies to control discomfort—everything from acupuncture to glucosamine/condroitin supplements to Tai Chi exercises to evening primrose oil. In many cases, we support trying various complementary therapies; a number of them truly seem to be helping large numbers of people feel better. Some of those therapies, however, have very little evidence to back them up, which is not surprising when you consider that they tend not to be put through the same rigorous testing as conventional treatments. Indeed, some can be harmful.

But it can be hard to distinguish what seems like a legitimate complementary therapy from the others. Advertising claims, word of mouth, and more lately Internet chat rooms have a way of making all of them sound equally helpful. For that reason, Chapter 9 describes some of the more popular complementary therapies that people with arthritis are hearing about today. For each one, we list the evidence (or lack thereof), the proposed mechanism of action, and all other pertinent information (including safety hazards). That way, you can make an informed decision about whether to try one of the treatments that does not have the official blessing of the medical community in the United States but that might just do you some good. Alternately, you will be alerted to those that have not shown any promise or, worse yet, could be detrimental to your health.

Joint replacement surgery

Perhaps you have been working with an arthritis specialist for years and also make an honest effort in trying all the suggestions we make in our program but still are extremely uncomfortable. Or maybe by the time you buy this book, your joint function has become compromised to the point that something more involved than lifestyle steps or medication is called for. That's when it might be time to consider joint replacement surgery.

But how do you find the right surgeon? How do you prepare for the surgery ahead of time so that you'll come out of it in the best shape possible? How much time should you plan to be off your feet? What about physical therapy? Are there drugs you should be taking—or discontinuing—before the operation? We answer these and many other questions regarding joint replacement so that in conjunction with your health-care professional, you can make the best decisions for the surgery and your recovery.

If you do opt for surgery, the program will still benefit you because improving your fitness (especially your strength) prior to the operation will only speed your recovery and improve the outcome. And the nutrition component may help you lose extra pounds that could make successful surgery go more smoothly and efficiently.

PUTTING IT ALL TOGETHER

It's not just that we *believe* the suggestions we make in this book will help you live a fuller life with less pain. We've *seen* it over and over again as we've worked with many different people. But while everything we advise is eminently doable, we don't mean to imply that it's a snap.

Lifestyle changes take a considerable amount of effort. You've got to shop somewhat differently, plan meals in a new way, carve out time for exercise—even when, during the first few weeks, you might not feel like doing it—and make a number of other adjustments to habits that may have become ingrained over many years. And it takes a certain leap of faith to do all that *before* the relief from pain starts to kick in (although in time it will).

The good news here is that we've broken down the lifestyle shifts into small steps that build on each other as you go along so that you won't feel overwhelmed by the process. We also devote a significant amount of discussion to the kinds of thought processes *behind* lifestyle changes—the ones that make them happen as well as those that keep them from happening. In fact, by going through the mental exercises in Chapter 6, you'll be able to see the emotional triggers in your own life that goad you on to better habits as well as the triggers that keep you stuck, so to speak, so you'll be equipped to "talk to yourself" in a way that will keep you progressing.

To help you maintain your inspiration as you go along, we've also included a workbook for you to chart your progress. Nothing motivates and keeps you on track like a written record: It's a terrific feeling to be able to tally up successes and movement forward. Seeing on paper the gaps in adherence that inevitably occur from time to time works as a good "shot in the arm," too.

At all points you'll understand *why* we make the recommendations we do. In Chapters 2 and 3 we explain not only how arthritis takes hold in the body but also discuss the specific research behind our advice. We included this information because we believe that knowledge is a powerful motivator. Knowledge of how your body works, in conjunction with knowledge of how to manipulate it to your best advantage, will allow you to be an active participant in your own health-care decisions, rather than a passive recipient of prescriptions and instructions.

Finally, there's a nuts-and-bolts resources section near the back of the book so that you can contact various organizations for information on everything from locating a doctor who specializes in arthritis to choosing exercise equipment to joining a support group.

Despite all the tools we offer, the changes that you make to take you out of pain are up to you—only *you* can do it. But you're not alone. Just as we were thrilled for the successes of the participants in our research, we are excited for you and the better life you're about to discover. And in that sense, just as with the volunteers we were lucky enough to meet in person and help toward more freedom of movement (not to mention a whole new outlook on life), we're with you every step of the way.

CHAPTER 2

Just What *Is* Arthritis?

■

There are about 120 places in the body where two bones come together in ways that allow movement. What that means, simply put, is that there are about 120 joints. Without the proper cushioning that joints provide, bones that meet would rub up against each other, making impossible all the normal movements of everyday living that most people take for granted. These movements include everything from gripping a pencil (there are 3 joints per finger) to taking a step, bending an elbow, and flexing toes.

Because you're reading this book, chances are that you—or someone important to you—already doesn't take certain movements for granted as a result of arthritis. Arthritis, quite literally, means joint disease (*arthro-* = *joint* and *-itis* = *inflammation*). The hallmark of this illness is breakdown of joint cartilage—the cushioning between two bones that acts as a shock absorber.

OSTEOARTHRITIS: THE MOST COMMON TYPE

There are more than one hundred different types of arthritis, and every type falls into one of two distinct categories: *degenerative* or *inflammatory*. The most prevalent type of degenerative arthritis by far is osteoarthritis, which accounts for about 80 percent of all arthritis and affects millions of people around the world. The most prevalent type of inflammatory arthritis is rheumatoid arthritis, which afflicts roughly one or two in one hundred people, or about 3–5 million Americans.

How joints work

If you've ever seen pictures of an active volcano, then you know how lava keeps spewing forth, spreading out beyond itself and forming land that wasn't there before. Think of the production of cartilage as you would a very slow lava flow. A layer of specialized cells called *chondrocytes* (the "volcanoes") slowly secrete a special cartilage gel (the "lava"). The cartilage gel is comprised of two different types of materials. One is *collagen*, which is akin to strong "ropes" and provides the cartilage its scaffolding. The other type of material in cartilage goes under the heading *proteoglycans*. These are little elasticized "springs" that connect the "ropes." They're crucial because they dam up water between them, providing the joint with elasticity and its ability to slide easily. Water also provides foolproof cushioning. It can't be compressed (think of a water balloon that you can't smush down), but it can easily be squeezed from place to place, which means it can even out the pressure in cartilage by flowing from an area of high pressure to an area of lower pressure (the same principle employed in many of the new "high-tech" soles in running shoes).

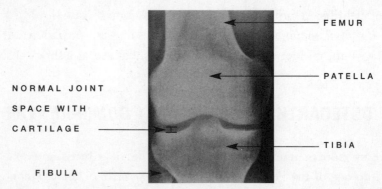

X-ray of a normal knee:
The bones of the joint, as pictured, include the femur, tibia, fibula, and patella (knee cap). The shadow between the femur and tibia represents the joint space, which includes the cartilage.

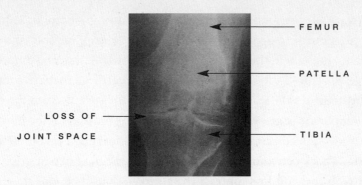

FEMUR

PATELLA

LOSS OF
JOINT SPACE

TIBIA

X-ray of a knee with osteoarthritis:

Notice the markedly reduced space between the femur and the tibia. This indicates a wearing away of the cartilage. In some places bone is rubbing against bone.

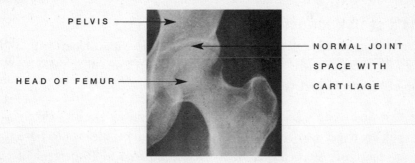

PELVIS

HEAD OF FEMUR

NORMAL JOINT
SPACE WITH
CARTILAGE

X-ray of a normal left hip:

The shadow between the head of the femur and the pelvis represents the joint space, which includes the cartilage.

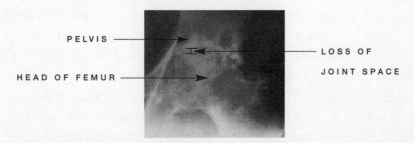

PELVIS

HEAD OF FEMUR

LOSS OF
JOINT SPACE

X-ray of a hip with osteoarthritis:

Notice the markedly reduced space between the head of the femur and the pelvis. Similar to the knee, this indicates a wearing away of the cartilage. In some places bone is rubbing against bone.

The process of distributing pressure throughout a joint works as follows: When you put a load on a joint, say, by walking or gripping something with your hand, muscles in the area move the bones, which in turn compress the cartilage. Specifically, it's the springs inside the cartilage that are compressing. This squeezes the water out from between the springs from the middle of the joint to the edges, which, in turn, allows the pressure of the movement to be evenly applied across the joint. After the movement is completed, the water flows back between the springs, ready for the next step or grip.

But with age, you lose some of the springs—and therefore some of the elasticity. The springs that remain become more brittle and less springy. In some people, the joint wear-and-tear of a lifetime (think of all the steps you have ever taken) leads to osteoarthritis; in others, it doesn't.

Who's at risk for osteoarthritis?

It can't be predicted with certainty who will end up with osteoarthritis and who will not. But there are definitely some risk factors that make some people more *prone* to developing the disease.

- *Age:* This is the biggest risk factor. The older you are, the more likely you are to get osteoarthritis. Roughly half of all people over 65 have evidence of osteoarthritis on X-rays (compared to 16 percent of people ages 18–44), and 10–15 percent of older adults have arthritis pain severe enough to require medication.
- *Gender:* One out of three women has the disease, compared with one out of four men. It's not yet clear, but it's suspected that there are hormonal influences that increase the risk for osteoarthritis in women. Indeed, in women approaching menopause, there's a tendency for osteoarthritis to develop in the joints of the knuckles that are closest to the fingertips. But most people, women and men alike, develop osteoarthritis in a large joint, such as in the knee or hip.
- *Excess weight:* The more you weigh, the more you stress the joints of the knees and hips. Consider that for every pound you carry on your frame, the pressure on the knees and hips increases by 3 pounds' worth as you walk. In other words, if you are 10 pounds overweight, your knees and hips experience the excess as if it were 30 pounds. The mechanism by which excess weight contributes to osteoarthri-

tis is not completely understood—it probably has to do with either
the increased wear and tear on the joint and/or hormonal factors.

- *Occupation:* Those whose jobs involve manual labor can spend years
  putting extra pressure on a particular joint or set of joints and can
  wear them out.
- *Injury:* Athletes and others who have injured their joints along the
  way are at increased risk (although moderate exercise appears to
  protect stressed joints).
- *Family history:* If your mother or father had osteoarthritis, you are
  more likely to develop it.
- *Muscle weakness:* If your muscles, especially your quadriceps (front
  of the thigh) and hamstrings (back of the thigh) are weak, you are at
  an elevated risk for developing osteoarthritis. This will be discussed
  in detail later in the chapter.

High heels—skinny or wide—can cost you your knees.

You might have figured that stiletto heels come with a health
price. After all, something that makes you look so great can't be
good for you.

You're right. Besides giving you bunions and crushed toes, high
heels worn on a habitual basis can set you up for osteoarthritis of
the knee. Researchers at Boston's Spaulding Rehabilitation Hospital
made the finding when they recorded the movements of 20 women
who frequently wore heels at least 2 inches high. The heels, it turned
out, increased torque (a twisting force) at the knee, straining the joint
near the back of the kneecap. They also strained the inner side of the
knee joint. Both of those stresses could eventually lead to enough
wear and tear to cause knee arthritis.

Unfortunately, switching to chunky high heels won't help. The
same team of researchers discovered, in fact, that chunky high heels
put even more pressure on women's knees than the stiletto kind.

Our advice: Toss the heels. Healthy is much sexier than disabled.

WHEN GOOD JOINTS GO BAD

Arthritis develops when stress on the joints causes small microcracks in cartilage that compromise the workings of the "ropes" and "springs." That's why osteoarthritis is often referred to as "wear-and-tear" arthritis. But to say that the disease develops solely from wear and tear is too simplistic. Today we know that the immune system is intimately involved. What happens is that the microcracks eventually gain the attention of the body's immune system, because it's the immune system's job to repair damaged areas. The problem is that the white cells of the immune system *cause* damage even as they clear it up: They carry enzymes that break down cartilage.

Furthermore, immune system or not, the ability of cartilage to repair itself is limited compared to the self-repairability to other areas of the body because there's no blood supply in cartilage to bathe it with nutrients that can help heal it. On one level that's a good thing. Without a blood supply and without a nerve supply that would go with it, pain is eliminated (which is why a healthy joint doesn't hurt when you use it). But the trade-off is that healing goes on much more slowly. Nutrients must enter the joints via diffusion from surrounding tissues rather than through direct infusion from the bloodstream.

The slow healing allows some of the microfractures to widen to the point that the cartilage cracks further—enough to be seen with the naked eye if you could see it under the skin. At the same time, the cartilage starts shrinking and losing some of its water content, and thus its "springiness," forming an ever thinning, ever more vulnerable layer of protection between the bones. Not only does that bring the bones closer together, it's also harder for a thinning joint to receive nourishment. Finally, the cartilage gets rough, like an unsanded surface—exactly the opposite from the way it should be. Consider that a normal, healthy joint is more slippery than ice on ice! But with arthritis, that smoothness is replaced by rough, cracked cartilage that snags and creaks.

In addition, the bones enlarge in order to spread the distribution of pressure. But they don't enlarge in a way that restores function. They form spurs, which can impede joint motion even more. The body, of course, sounds an alert to these changes with pain. Where does the pain come from if the cartilage doesn't have any nerve endings? It comes from bone, from the joint capsule that surrounds the joint, and from tendons and ligaments, all of which have nerve endings.

The more pain, the less you're likely to use a joint. This disuse, along with joint inflammation, causes atrophy of the muscle surrounding the joint. Therein lies one of the biggest difficulties with osteoarthritis—as well as one of the solutions to the problem.

The role of muscle

Cartilage in the joint cushions bones and keeps them from banging into each other. But something else cushions the bones as well—muscle. In fact, muscle is the most important protector of joints; cartilage only absorbs shock

Who's your doctor?

If you have joint pain, you should see your primary care doctor first. For most patients with osteoarthritis, the primary care doctor is all you'll need. If you have rheumatoid or another kind of inflammatory arthritis, or severe osteoarthritis, you may need to see a rheumatologist. A rheumatologist is an internist who has had 2–3 additional years of training in the diagnosis and treatment of arthritis, lupus, and other connective tissue diseases.

Your doctor or specialist may order X-rays, blood tests, bone density scans, or other tests to diagnose your arthritis. Common blood tests include one for sedimentation rate, which tells about whole-body inflammation, and one for rheumatoid factor, a test that is positive in three-quarters of patients with rheumatoid arthritis.

As a patient, you must speak up if you're confused, uncertain, scared, or in pain. Don't expect your doctor to read your mind—take the initiative and ask questions! How else can you be confident that you are being treated properly?

that gets *past* the muscle. It's for that reason that muscle weakness is so bad for joints. Without strong muscle, cartilage wears out much sooner!

To understand how cartilage and muscle work together, think of a car going over bumps. It's the job of the car's shock absorbers to take each bump as it comes and not send a jarring shock up to the passengers. If they fail, the car's springs and axles take the shock, but the passengers really feel that and may even hear it! In your body, the muscles are the shock absorbers, and the cartilage is the spring and axle assembly. Most of the time, when you walk or run, your muscles absorb the brunt of the shock so your joints don't have to. But once in a while, if you aren't looking or if you trip or step off a curb wrong, you may feel a painful shock in your knee. Researchers call that a *microklutz,* and it means that the shock got past your muscles and hit your cartilage, sending a pain signal through the bone and nerves to your brain. Over many years, such shocks can slowly degrade the cartilage.

As arthritis develops with cartilage degradation, pain forces people to use their joints less. But when you don't use your joints, you're not using your muscles, and they weaken. And that leads to a damaged joint absorbing even more trauma with every motion; the muscles just can't do the job they're supposed to. The result, in turn, is that damage to the joint accelerates, setting in motion a vicious cycle: pain → inactivity → muscle weakness → joint damage → more pain, and the cycle repeats itself.

The good news is that while you can't grow new cartilage to replace cartilage that has worn away, you *can* grow new muscle and thereby rebuild a critical part of the joints' shock-absorbing system. It might seem counterintuitive to exercise a muscle in the part of the body where there's arthritis pain. But in Chapter 4 we'll show you how to work around it—safely and comfortably—to the point that the pain lessens and you have more freedom of movement than you may have had in years.

RHEUMATOID ARTHRITIS: A DISEASE OF MANY JOINTS

If you have osteoarthritis, there might be just one affected joint—the knee joint, perhaps, or the hip joint. In the case of rheumatoid arthritis, however, the action of as many as 20–30 joints may be compromised. Moreover, it's a

Arthritis affects the mind as well as the body.

Arthritis causes much more than loss of easy mobility. The pain can be unrelenting, which in turn can lead to loss of sleep. Indeed, according to at least one study conducted at the University of North Carolina at Chapel Hill, sleep disruption outweighs more obvious arthritis concerns, including reduced ability to get around, missed work, and inability to participate in favorite recreational activities.

It's not just pain that inhibits sleep, at least in people with rheumatoid arthritis. Body chemicals involved in that form of the disease work directly on brain chemicals that control the ability to slumber. They're called *cytokines*, and besides contributing to inflammation of the joints, they change brain "excitability" and thereby alter sleep patterns. Restorative REM sleep is lost, and there's much more awakening through the night.

On top of the lack of sleep, arthritis pain can cause depression. In fact, depression is one of the hallmarks of the disease. And it doesn't have anything to do with whether you have a sunny or gloomy disposition to start with. It, too, is physiological—any kind of chronic pain will lead to a chemical stress response in the brain. And that stress is interpreted as depression. The depression may not be severe, and the patient may not recognize it, but psychological testing does show it in a very high proportion of people with arthritis. Others develop irritability, anxiety, or inability to concentrate.

The chemical aspect of these changes in mood and outlook has to do with the fact that the brain contains a network of *neurotransmitters*, packets of chemicals that work to signal our emotions and thoughts between brain cells. Normally, there's a balance between excitatory and inhibitory neurotransmitters. But with any chronic stress, that balance gets out of whack. On top of that, there really *is* a reason to feel depressed. Pain, sleep deprivation, and loss of mobility do not make for a bright outlook.

It might seem that if you could get the pain of arthritis under control, the depression would automatically dissipate. But it doesn't necessarily work that way. That's because if the depression has been present for a while, it *changes* the brain's chemical makeup, and that may require separate treatment in the form of therapy and/or antidepressant medication. Thus, if you feel like you're not getting pleasure out of life, even after you've effectively reduced arthritis pain, you may need to address the depression head-on. Going for some therapy or counseling is an option, as is treatment with antidepressant medication. Research in our laboratory at Tufts has shown that exercise on its own is also effective at reducing at least mild to moderate depression and improving self-confidence. The more confident you are, the better you feel about yourself.

disease that involves the whole body, changing the body's metabolism and involving the immune system in all the tissues, not just those in the joints. That's why, unlike osteoarthritis, rheumatoid arthritis is called a *systemic disease*—it affects every system in the body.

Certainly, almost any joint, large or small, can be affected with rheumatoid arthritis, but usually it's the small joints of the hands and feet that are most severely compromised. Wherever the disease strikes, its damage to the joints occurs much faster, much more aggressively, than the damage of osteoarthritis. And it can be much more crippling. After 20 years with rheumatoid arthritis, about half of patients are disabled, and the death rate in people with the disease is double that of healthy people the same age. Furthermore, unlike osteoarthritis, which occurs in middle-aged and older adults, rheumatoid arthritis is not a disease of aging. It can occur from about age 2 on.

At Tufts, we believe a lot of the disability and mortality is due to loss of muscle induced by the inflammation, which is why preservation of muscle through exercise is so important.

If your child has Juvenile Chronic Arthritis

Arthritis has no respect for age. While degenerative forms of arthritis such as osteoarthritis are almost nonexistent in children, even those under 2 years of age can—and do—develop inflammatory arthritis. Formerly called *Juvenile Rheumatoid Arthritis*, it is now referred to as *Juvenile Chronic Arthritis*, and it comes in many forms, similar to the various types of adult inflammatory arthritis.

Rheumatologists classify Juvenile Chronic Arthritis based on the number of joints affected. It can be monoarticular, involving just a single joint; pauciarticular, involving three or fewer joints; or polyarticular, affecting more than three joints. Depending on the number of joints involved and the specific form of the disease, there will be differences in response to treatment, in the prognosis for future mobility, and in the risk for developing complications outside the joints, such as in the eyes and skin (Juvenile Chronic Arthritis can cause vision loss, or even blindness, and can also cause many types of rashes).

Today most children can be treated very effectively, but treatment can be tricky. Juvenile Chronic Arthritis can stunt growth, as can some of the medications used to treat it, especially steroids such as prednisone. To complicate matters further, children are not usually studied in clinical trials of new treatments, so it can be years before it is clear whether a new medicine is safe or effective for youngsters.

Of course, seeing a child with joint pain and difficulty moving is painful for any parent. But treatment inroads *are* being made, and today, both treatment and prognosis for a freer-moving, less painful future are better than they were even 10 years ago. Indeed, even with various problems with drugs, the development of new medications has revolutionized the care of children with arthritis and prevented crippling deformities that were once inevitable in children with the disease.

Treatment is highly specialized, however, and children with Juvenile

Chronic Arthritis should be seen by a board-certified rheumatologist and, if possible, a pediatric rheumatologist, on a regular basis. To find a pediatric rheumatologist in your area, contact your local chapter of the Arthritis Foundation (see "Resources" at the back of the book for contact information). With proper care children with Juvenile Chronic Arthritis can look forward to full and normal lives.

How rheumatoid arthritis takes its toll

In people with rheumatoid arthritis, the immune system attacks the body's own tissues, which means the condition is an autoimmune disease. The joints are what initially undergo the attack. Specifically, the *synovium,* a membrane that surrounds the entire joint, is invaded by a huge number of white blood cells. The white blood cell invasion is what causes the warmth, redness, swelling, and pain—in a word, the inflammation. The white cells also break down collagen and bone, in part by producing high levels of "free radicals"—bullet-like atoms of oxygen and hydrogen that kill bacteria. But in rheumatoid arthritis they damage joints instead.

Worse still, the white blood cells replace the synovium with a destructive mass of blood vessels and other cells called *pannus.* Pannus is much thicker than the synovium itself, which contributes to the stiffness felt by those with rheumatoid arthritis. That thickness also doesn't allow nutrients to get through to the joint. Healthy synovium is only one or two cell layers thick, which makes it thin enough to allow the entry of various vitamins, along with glucose (the basic component of carbohydrates), amino acids (the basic components of protein), fats, and oxygen. But because pannus is hundreds of cells thick, the joint becomes malnourished and less capable of repairing any damage.

To make matters even worse, all of the activity by the white cells of the immune system rev up metabolism, putting the body on overdrive. And that, in turn, causes muscle wasting.

Rheumatoid arthritis and muscle deterioration

The body's mass is divided into two parts—fat and lean. The lean mass is further divided four ways: muscle, bone, viscera (internal organs), and the immune system. In a healthy person, metabolic rate—or the number of calories burned each day—is determined almost entirely by the amount of muscle and viscera present. Fat, bone, and the immune system have virtually nothing to do with metabolism or calorie burning.

But in someone with rheumatoid arthritis, the immune system is working so hard that it does change metabolism. Indeed, in someone with rheumatoid arthritis, metabolism speeds up by about 20 percent—a possible cause of a lot of the fatigue associated with the condition.

Of course, if the metabolic rate is up by 20 percent, that means 20 percent more calories are required. Where do they come from? Unfortunately, they do not come from the body's fat stores, which would be the "logical" place. They come from stores of lean tissue that make up muscle, which is comprised largely of protein. It's protein that makes up the components of the overcharged immune system: white blood cells, antibodies, and so on. Thus, protein calories burned by the immune system are the type that have to get replaced. The immune system itself sets this up. Specifically, when the immune system becomes activated in rheumatoid arthritis, it secretes cytokines, chemical signals in the body that change the mix of what the body burns for fuel from predominantly fat and carbohydrates to one that includes much more protein and a lot less fat. The protein that is needed to fuel the immune system comes from its storage depot—muscle.

The wearing down of muscle protein to "re-stock" the immune system is dramatic. Normally, when people reach their seventies, they have about 20 percent less muscle than they did in their twenties. That's typical aging in a healthy person. But our research at Tufts shows that people with rheumatoid arthritis have much greater than average muscle loss. What it comes down to is that a 70-year-old with the disease has about one-third less muscle than a healthy 25-year-old. Considering that people die when they lose about 40 percent of the muscle mass they have in young adulthood, it's easy to see why people with rheumatoid arthritis have a mortality rate that is two to five times greater than that of the general population.

Unfortunately, you can't eat your way out of the muscle loss. That is, eating a lot of calories in the form of protein won't help. The protein simply gets burned to fuel the immune system, and if the protein provides any excess calories, they turn (frustratingly) to fat, not muscle. Indeed, even while their revved metabolisms burn so many calories, people with rheumatoid arthritis are more likely than others to store fat.

Ironically, with all that fat accumulation, people with rheumatoid arthritis don't necessarily gain much weight. Instead, what often happens is that body weight stays the same, but the proportion of muscle to fat drops significantly. So the arthritis sufferer, without gaining a pound, becomes overfat with poor muscle tone. And because of the pain and weakness, physical activity is reduced, causing further muscle atrophy. The upshot: a higher risk for heart disease and stroke—all the problems associated with too much body fat and too little muscle. But it is possible to regain this muscle, as you will see in Chapter 3.

Other types of inflammatory arthritis

Rheumatoid arthritis is just one type of inflammatory arthritis. Granted, it's the one that's studied most—probably more than half of all people who have inflammatory arthritis have this kind. However, our program for reversing arthritis pain and disability should be effective for mitigating the effects of other types of inflammatory arthritis, too, including some of the more common ones mentioned here.

Lupus

Systemic lupus erythematosis, as it is known in medical circles, is an autoimmune disease that can affect any part of the body. Called "lupus" because it can cause a rash that scars and looked to nineteenth-century doctors like a wolf bite (*lupus* is Latin for wolf), it most commonly affects young women. There are limited forms of lupus that affect only the skin, but more aggressive lupus can affect the brain, blood vessels, lungs, heart, abdomen, and nervous system.

Sjögren's syndrome

This is a combination of dry mouth and dry eyes. Less commonly, people with this syndrome develop other autoimmune symptoms, such as joint pain, nerve damage, and liver disease. However, most people "just" have the dry eyes and mouth, which are uncomfortable but not dangerous. They are treated with artificial tears and urged to drink lots of fluids, but the symptoms can sometimes be difficult to control. Sjögren's syndrome can also cause problems (blockages) of the arteries. The most dangerous aspect of Sjögren's syndrome is an increased risk for lymphoma, or cancer of the lymph glands. Lymphoma is ten to forty times more common in people with Sjögren's than in others, but, even so, that complication is quite rare.

Ankylosing spondylitis, Reiter's syndrome, psoriatic arthritis,
and arthritis of inflammatory bowel disease

These four conditions are collectively called the *seronegative spondyloarthropathies* or *rheumatoid variants,* medical mouthfuls that simply mean inflammatory arthritis that is not rheumatoid arthritis. The common thread in all of these is arthritis involving many joints, usually including those in the spine, hips, and knees.

Unlike rheumatoid arthritis, the seronegative arthritic diseases do not have a positive blood test for rheumatoid factor. Also, unlike rheumatoid arthritis, these diseases do not respond to low doses of steroids like prednisone or to gold. They are treated more often with sulfasalazine or methotrexate, two drugs that are effective in treating rheumatoid arthritis (discussed in more detail in Chapter 7). Tissues that can be affected by ankylosing spondylitis include the lungs, heart, and eyes.

Gout

Gout is the major type of inflammatory arthritis in men. It is caused by a buildup of uric acid, a normal by-product of protein and DNA metabolism. Some people produce too much uric acid, and others have a minor kidney defect that prevents them from excreting it properly in the urine. Typically, gout causes arthritis flares of one or a few joints that are extremely severe but generally go away within 7–10 days. Over time, the attacks can get longer and eventually merge into a continuous painful arthritis called *chronic gout,*

which can destroy the joints as severely as rheumatoid arthritis. Before effective treatment became available in the 1950s, half of those with gout became
disabled within 20 years of diagnosis. And since most patients are men in
their thirties or forties when they are diagnosed, this was a major problem.
Nowadays, however, there is no reason for gout to progress to this level of
severity; the disease can be controlled in all but the most extreme cases.

Pseudogout

This is the "other" type of inflammatory arthritis caused by deposition of a
chemical in the joint. But instead of uric acid (the typical cause in gout), the
culprit here is calcium phosphate, the same stuff that makes up bone.

In most cases a milder disease than gout, pseudogout most often affects
the wrists, elbows, and knees, and is most common in elderly women. Unlike
gout, pseudogout is not crippling, even though it can be quite painful and is
often tricky to diagnose. This disease, too, can be effectively controlled with
medication.

Lyme disease

Lyme disease is an infectious arthritis caused by a bacteria called *Borrelia
bergdorferi*. This germ is carried by deer ticks and is found in areas where deer
are common, including the Northeast and Middle Atlantic states, Wisconsin,
and parts of Europe. It usually causes only a single bout of arthritis at the
time of infection and can be cured with antibiotics in most patients. However,
there are some people who are genetically predisposed to developing chronic
arthritis after infection with Lyme disease. In those cases, it usually causes
chronic arthritis of one or two joints. Lyme disease can also cause damage to
the heart, brain, and skin.

Vasculitis

Vasculitis means "inflammation of the blood vessels." This condition leads to
swelling of the arteries and blockage of blood flow, which in turn causes
damage to the organs supplied by the affected blood vessels. The lungs,
heart, brain, gastrointestinal tract, nerves, and muscles can be affected. Note
that vasculitis, as well as lupus, can sometimes lead to cognitive, or brain-
functioning, changes that make it difficult to concentrate and execute high-
order mental skills, such as mathematics. Memory can be impaired, too. Often,

there's no specific treatment for these brain changes, but people with these conditions should be aware of them so they don't think they're "losing it."

Fibromyalgia

Fibromyalgia is a cluster of symptoms that includes pain in many areas of the body, poor sleep, and often mood disorders, and it affects women much more commonly than men. The pain, often in the back, arms, and legs, usually occurs in muscular areas, rather than in the joints themselves. There is no evidence of inflammation by any objective measure. In fact, fibromyalgia is very poorly understood and may last for years. Many physicians do not believe that it is a distinct disease. They feel that it is a manifestation of depression or other psychological illness. Others disagree, pointing to the common features of the disease and its high prevalence. Although fibromyalgia causes a great deal of long-term pain, it does not cripple or deform joints. There is little useful treatment, other than low doses of antidepressants and exercise. Several studies have shown that exercise improves fibromyalgia, although often there is a transient worsening for the first six weeks or so. If you have fibromyalgia, we suggest you try our program slowly and carefully, and limit yourself to twice-weekly exercise for the first six weeks before starting the program fully.

MORE THAN A SILVER LINING

It's true that while nobody dies of arthritis, people with the disease are much more likely than healthy adults to feel sick, become disabled, and develop secondary illnesses due to inactivity, obesity, and loss of muscle. But scientists have made tremendous strides in the past decade in learning how arthritis works—and how to block it. New medications have transformed the ability of physicians to control inflammation, which retards muscle loss; and new devices and techniques have made it possible to replace joints that have been damaged beyond salvage, as you will learn in Chapter 8.

Of course, while they can prevent more damage to joints, these new treatments don't regenerate muscle or rehabilitate people so they can regain function after their arthritis has come under control. That's where this book comes in. Our goal is to return people to optimal function and health. To do this, we will show you the lifestyle steps you can take on your own to give your muscles the stimulus they need to grow, strengthen, and protect your joints while making you more independent—and reducing your pain.

Our program is the natural extension of the medical treatment that your physician, nurse, and physical therapist may have already started. But, unlike their ministrations, *you* are the key ingredient in our program. If you work at it, we are confident that you will see powerful results that will surprise and delight you.

CHAPTER 3

The Science Behind the Program

■

Although some kinds of arthritis have been found in Egyptian mummies, and Hypocrites described joint swelling and pain, arthritis only began to be discussed in scientific terms about 125 years ago. In 1876, a British scientist named James Paget described a condition that he called *rheumatoid cachexia* (*rheumatoid*, meaning "pain and swelling," and *cachexia*, meaning "wasting"). In other words, he was describing the wasting of the muscles and the painful joints that accompany arthritis. But for 100 years after that, the prescribed treatment for arthritis was rest. Doctors thought that the best way to help the joints retain their function was not to move them.

EARLY PROOF THAT EXERCISE BRINGS BENEFITS

Researchers didn't begin to look seriously at the beneficial effects of exercise on arthritis until the mid-1970s. In 1974, a study showed that moving the joints through exercise improved arthritis—or at least kept it from getting worse. Exercise appeared to mitigate pain as well. But the study, conducted in Sweden and published in a Scandanavian journal, received scant attention in the United States.

In fact, from the mid-1970s through the 1990s, researchers in the United States as well as in other countries made only sporadic efforts to test the notion that exercise could help reduce the pain and disability of arthritis by increasing the strength of the muscles that support the joints.

In all, about a dozen reasonably well-controlled studies were conducted. On the whole, they suggested that exercise helps people with arthritis but concluded that its effect was modest at best. Part of the reason for these lukewarm findings was that some of the studies did not focus on the types of exercise that we now know form the cornerstone of a solid exercise program for people with the disease.

Why aerobics alone fell short

Several investigative efforts suggested that aerobic activities like walking may have a modest effect on the pain and disability associated with osteoarthritis of the knee. But those studies had an inherent problem in that, for people with moderate to severe knee arthritis, walking can be extremely painful. Indeed, it's an activity that people with knee arthritis often *avoid*.

Just as important, walking, unlike weight lifting or strength training, does not address the muscle weakness that has so much to do with arthritis pain and disability. So it doesn't really get to the heart of the problem. It's not that walking is not a good activity for many people with arthritis, but starting a walking program before engaging in an exercise program to strengthen the muscles supporting the knees and hips is doing things backward.

Why the first look at strength training was less than encouraging

While some of the early research focused on aerobics such as walking, about a dozen other studies did, in fact, focus on strength training, or resistance training. The results were inconsistent, however.

Take, for example, the largest of these studies—the Fitness Arthritis and Seniors Trial (FAST), conducted at the Bowman Gray School of Medicine at Wake Forest University in North Carolina. More than four hundred men and women were assigned either to a strength-training program, a walking program, or a health education program without any exercise at all. Eighteen months later, the two exercise groups were doing better than the health-education group, but not by much. They experienced only about 8–10 percent less pain and disability—a change that was due more to the fact that the non-exercisers got worse than to an actual improvement in their symptoms as a result of the exercises. That is, the exercise prevented a further decline but caused few, if any, improvements. Of course, preventing further decline has value in and of itself, but we here at Tufts wondered whether it might be possible to get much *more* out of a strength-training program. We had reason to believe it would. Why? When we scrutinized the FAST study, we found that the people who had engaged in strength training did not get much stronger. And that was a clue that the exercises hadn't gone far enough, that they weren't intense enough. When you strength-train properly by lifting weights or using resistance machines, your muscles become more powerful. That's the whole point.

Thus, we reasoned, if the "dose" of exercise prescribed had been a little larger, with more of an effort to specifically target weak muscles, the strength training would not have simply prevented a decline in arthritis symptoms. It would have actually caused an improvement, allowing people to regain a level of comfort and mobility that they had lost. We certainly had hints of that from other studies we conducted at Tufts.

WHAT THE TUFTS UNIVERSITY RESEARCH FOUND

Our studies here at Tufts University have shown that older people who engage in aggressive strength-training programs that truly target and challenge their muscles improve their strength and function to the level of people decades younger. The older volunteers in our strength-training studies can once again run up and down the stairs with a pile of laundry and not get winded, lift heavy packages with more ease, and go through the day with more energy. In one study that Miriam conducted with colleagues, it was found that older women who strength-trained at the proper intensity even strengthened their bones to the point of reducing their risk for osteoporosis.

As a result of the success of these studies, Ronenn Roubenoff decided to investigate whether strength training could help people with arthritis. He and another Tufts researcher, Laura Rall, Ph.D., demonstrated that people with rheumatoid arthritis who engaged regularly in appropriate strength-training exercises actually *reversed* the muscle weakness that proves so devastating to people with that disease. Participants in this study felt so much better because of the exercises they were doing at the laboratory that they could participate in social and sports activities they hadn't been able to engage in for years.

Up until this point, all of our exercise programs had been conducted right at our Tufts laboratory. But we wanted to see if people could follow strength-training programs on their own. After all, not everybody can come into a laboratory—or even go to a health club for that matter. It was that interest, and our strong desire to lessen arthritis symptoms, that led to the definitive research behind our program.

The definitive Tufts study

We joined forces to develop a research project that would look at the effect of strength training on older adults with osteoarthritis of the knee—*in their own homes.* It was a novel concept because all the past related studies had been conducted at research facilities with strength-training equipment—and with experts who could provide one-on-one training for study subjects at every single exercise session. This new research would leave people more on their own.

Getting funding to try new ideas isn't always easy. Fortunately, the Medical Foundation in Boston, a nonprofit association whose mission is to foster research on strategies for helping older adults to live independently, was at that time requesting grant applications to fund a study on how adults could remain active participants in their own communities. We applied for that grant—specifically to see if people with osteoarthritis of the knee could improve their ability to live independently by building stronger muscles via strength training—and received it.

The nuts and bolts of the Tufts research

Once the funding was in place, Kristin, a doctoral student at Tufts at the time, joined our efforts. We recruited forty-six arthritis sufferers who experienced pain almost every day and thus were significantly limited in their ability to participate in the normal activities of daily life—walking, stair climbing, even just sitting and standing. Then Kristin went to each of their homes several times throughout the course of the four-month study.

Half of the people completed a 16-week strength-training program whose intensity was designed to increase muscle strength rather than just put people through a range of motions. The other half simply received emotional support from Kristin: She gave them attention and provided some general guidelines about a healthful diet (*not* a diet geared toward diminishing arthritis pain). This group was the control group, and they were crucial to the study because previous research had shown that even receiving attention can improve the symptoms of osteoarthritis to some degree. We wanted to separate out improvements due to strength training from improvements that resulted from the increased attention of a visiting researcher.

The exercise group didn't use any of the elaborate equipment you would find in a research lab or even a gym. They worked with simple, inexpensive equipment like ankle weights. Even staircases and chairs in their homes served as "equipment" for certain exercise routines—and the results were remarkable!

"Eureka —I am stronger and have less pain!"

After the 4 months were up, pain in the exercise group decreased by an average of 43 percent as opposed to only 12 percent in the placebo group. And physical function improved by 44 percent overall in the exercise group— almost twice as much as in the placebo group. It was no wonder; the strength of the large muscles in the front of the thigh (quadriceps) near the afflicted knee increased an average of 71 percent! The exercisers were able to walk, climb stairs, sit, and stand more easily. And they slept more restfully. Improvements were actually seen in seventeen physical tasks of daily living, including going shopping, putting on socks and shoes, and getting out of a chair. Their entire lives turned around. All of a sudden, people who had found life's daily activities more and more challenging and painful as a result of arthritis pain were able to participate in life in ways they hadn't been able to for years.

The changes were even more astounding when you consider that up until this study was completed, the *only* treatments known to have a significant impact on the pain and disability suffered by people with osteoarthritis of the knee were joint replacement and drug regimens.

The benefits go beyond increased strength

Strength training does more than increase muscle strength. It has been clinically shown to reduce anxiety, boost self-confidence, and lift depression—all of which have been shown to directly impact a person's levels of both pain and disability.

In addition, strength training goes a long way in weight management—an important point, since the more overweight someone is, the more disabling the arthritis. Strength training helps reduce weight by increasing muscle mass: The more muscle you have, the more calories you end up burning to maintain that muscle. Simply put, your metabolism goes into high gear to burn excess body fat.

Strength-train even if you need surgery

Strength training is also beneficial for people who eventually come to need a joint replaced. Joint replacement surgery is only as successful as the condition of a person's musculature to begin with. Thus, if you go into knee replacement literally weak-kneed, you'll come out with much less pain and much more ability to get around, but there will still be limitations. If you regularly strength-train, on the other hand, and then have to have surgery down the line to replace a knee joint, you'll be able to make much better use of the new joint afterward because the muscles it uses to function will be in the best shape possible. In other words, the stronger and better your muscle function prior to surgery, the better the outcome *after* surgery.

THE INFLUENCE OF DIET ON ARTHRITIS

Not getting enough exercise—or the right type of exercise—is only one factor that may be contributing to the development of arthritis and to arthritis pain. Over the last two decades we have also learned an enormous amount about how *diet* impacts arthritis, in both positive and negative ways.

The dietary recommendations for controling the symptoms of arthritis are pretty much the same whether you have osteoarthritis or rheumatoid arthritis, but the *research* tends to break out into studies that look at the two diseases separately. That's why we describe that research in two separate sections here.

THE CONNECTION BETWEEN DIET AND OSTEOARTHRITIS

Four vitamins for osteoarthritis

The case for vitamin C

About 20 years ago, the Framingham Osteoarthritis Study came out of the now famous Framingham Heart Study. In 1983, residents of Framingham, Massachusetts, who had been observed for heart disease risk factors since 1948, began to be observed for their risk of developing osteoarthritis. What the researchers found was that the progression of osteoarthritis was reduced by more than half in people who consumed an average of at least 152 milligrams of vitamin C a day (almost twice the recommended amount). In people who had no pain but still had osteoarthritis on X-ray, the vitamin C protected against the development of knee pain in the future.

Vitamin C is thought to help reduce pain for two reasons. First, it is important in the formation of collagen and proteoglycans—the major components of cartilage. Second, it's an antioxidant nutrient that can quench free radicals. Free radicals—highly reactive and unstable compounds produced in the body—can rip through cartilage like bullets, damaging its structure. As the damage occurs, there's inflammation at the joint. People tend to think of inflammation as something that occurs only in cases of rheumatoid arthritis, but inflammation is involved in osteoarthritis, too. It's part of an immune response in cartilage to try to "deactivate" the free radicals and repair damage to the joint. That's where vitamin C is believed to be beneficial; it's thought to neutralize free radicals before they have a chance to destroy cartilage.

The case for vitamin D

Other findings from the Framingham Study showed that vitamin D is also important. Those people with knee arthritis who took in fewer than 350 International Units (IU) of vitamin D a day had a three- to four-fold greater risk for disease progression than those who consumed on the order of 400 IU or more per day (an amount that is difficult to get in your diet unless you drink a quart of milk a day).

How could vitamin D play a role? Osteoarthritis damages not just the cartilage but also the underlying bones. That's a problem because bones help maintain joint stability. Bones and cartilage "communicate" with each other to allow for a healthy joint. So any bone abnormalities resulting from osteoarthritis can contribute to loss of mobility. The way vitamin D comes into play here is that it's crucial for bone strength and structure. Indeed, in the Framingham population, people who had low levels of vitamin D in the blood were more likely to develop bone spurs.

Vitamin D is also believed to play a direct role in the cartilage itself, in chondrocytes. The chondrocytes produce collagen and proteoglycans, and there is some evidence that vitamin D may affect this function. Again, those in Framingham who had low blood levels of vitamin D were more likely to suffer the loss of cartilage, major components of which are collagen and proteoglycans.

The case for beta-carotene and vitamin E

The case for beta-carotene and vitamin E, both antioxidants, is not as strong as it is for vitamins C or D. Still, we feel that the research results to date, while preliminary, make a strong enough case that beta-carotene and vitamin E should at least be dietary *concerns* for people with osteoarthritis. The Framingham researchers did find that people with osteoarthritis of the knee who consumed more than 9,000 IU of beta-carotene a day (an amount easily obtained from a diet rich in fruits and vegetables) were at reduced risk for disease progression compared to people whose daily consumption was less than 5,000 IU. They were also much less likely to suffer knee pain down the line. Currently, because they eat very few fruits and vegetables, Americans are estimated to take in only 3,000–5,000 IU of beta-carotene each day.

As for vitamin E, people with knee arthritis in the Framingham trial who consumed 6–11 milligrams of vitamin E daily were 60 percent less likely over a 10-year period to experience disease progression than those who took in only 2–5 milligrams. Higher dosages—the type for which you'd need supplements rather than foods alone—did not increase protection.

However, a couple of studies conducted in Germany have suggested that supplementation with doses of vitamin E beyond what the diet can provide might be of help. In the study that was most rigorously controlled, fifty patients with osteoarthritis were given either 400 milligrams of vitamin E daily for 6 weeks or a placebo. Pain at rest was reduced twice as much in the vitamin E takers as in the placebo group. Pain upon moving around was also cut dramatically more in the vitamin E group than in the placebo group.

In another study, 400 milligrams of vitamin E a day was compared to the anti-inflammatory analgesic diclofenac (Voltaren) taken at doses of 50 milligrams, three times a day. The treatments were equally effective at reducing pain and improving joint mobility, but one in four people on diclofenac reported side effects such as stomach upset or heartburn, while only one in fourteen of those on vitamin E experienced side effects.

A weighty influence on joints

Every time you take a step, the force, or pressure, across your knees and hips is two to three times your body weight. When you're walking down stairs or rising from a chair, the pressure is even greater—six times your body weight. What does that mean in practical terms?

- If you weigh 150 pounds, when you walk, your knees and hips are shouldering the burden of closer to 450 pounds—a particular handicap for someone whose joints, or shock absorbers, have undergone significant deterioration.
- For the same 150-pound person, climbing down the front stoop is akin to putting up to 900 pounds of pressure on the knee joints!

Put another way, if you gain just 20 excess pounds, your knees carry a burden of up to *120* extra pounds. Of course, the more weight, the more pressure, the more pain—and the more joint deterioration. Excess weight can even adversely affect a person's gait, resulting in even *more* pressure on the joints. Extra weight doesn't just have the potential to exacerbate the symptoms of osteoarthritis—it appears to be a *cause* of the disease.

It used to be thought that weight gain *resulted* from osteoarthritis: The pain and disability accompanying knee arthritis in particular were believed to lead to a decline in physical activity and a subsequent putting on of pounds. While that's true, it is now clear that it's also largely the other way around. Studies in which people were followed *prior* to the onset of osteoarthritis have found that over time, being overweight increases the risk for joint problems later on in life. In research conducted at the Harvard School of Public Health, for instance, women who were overweight were four times as likely as women who weighed less to develop knee arthritis. Women who were considered medically obese were *ten* times as likely to go on to develop osteoarthritis of the knee.

What's the difference between overweight and obese? Health professionals use cutoff points according to people's body mass index, or BMI, which is a measure of weight for height. A BMI of up to 25 is considered healthy weight, while a BMI of 26–29 is overweight, and a BMI of 30 or greater, obese. Unfortunately, once someone develops osteoarthritis, the inactivity that often ensues as a result of the pain leads to even more weight gain—which only exacerbates the problem by leading to even more pain. It's a vicious cycle.

The good news in all of this is that you don't have to become model thin to cope with osteoarthritis. On the contrary, a small weight loss can make a very big difference in mitigating pain.

The ten-pound loss that can give you your life back

In conducting the Framingham osteoarthritis study, researchers found that a weight loss of just 2 units of BMI—which for most people amounts to about 11 pounds—decreased the risk for pain and stiffness by 50 percent! Gaining that much weight increased the severity of symptoms by the same amount. The glass-half-full side of that equation is that even maintaining weight, rather than gaining, can do a lot to prevent unnecessary pain.

It was a similar story with a study in Japan. A group of people with osteoarthritis who lost an average of 9 pounds in 6 weeks reported feeling less

Overweight women at greater risk for osteoarthritis than overweight men

Women who carry around excess weight are more likely than overweight men to end up with osteoarthritis. Researchers suspect it has something to do with hormonal differences between the sexes. How those differences come into play has not yet been sorted out, but it *is* known that too much body fat changes levels of various hormones that may result in an adverse effect on cartilage and bone.

Supporting the hormone-arthritis speculation is that the more excess poundage, the higher the risk appears to be for osteoarthritis of the hand, which cannot be chalked up simply to the mechanics of the way the hand moves with extra weight. Yes, more fat in the hands may exert greater force across the joints as the hand contracts, say, to grip a pencil. But in the Harvard study that looked at BMI and the risk for knee arthritis, the risk for osteoarthritis of the hand among women with a BMI of 28 or more was, on average, eight times greater than the risk among women whose BMI was less than 24. Such a dramatic difference cannot be attributed solely to the pressure of the extra weight on the joints.

For osteoarthritis of the hip, the Harvard researchers found that the risk is two to three times greater for women with a BMI over 24 compared to women with lower BMIs—again, too much of a difference to be accounted for solely by the force of weight across the hip.

pain and a greater ability to function than a similar group of people who did not lose the weight.

It makes sense that such relatively small amounts of weight could make such a big difference. Remember we said that for every pound you weigh, the force across your knees as you walk is up to three times that amount. Losing 10–11 pounds means taking about 30 pounds of pressure off the knees as

Body Mass Index (for Women and Men)

1. Read down the first column to locate your height.
2. Read across that row and locate your weight.
3. Read the heading on top of the column—that's your BMI.

UNDERWEIGHT BMI under 19		HEALTHY WEIGHT BMI 19–25							OVERWEIGHT BMI 26–29			
HEIGHT (inches)	18 or less	19	20	21	22	23	24	25	26	27	28	29
58	86	91	96	100	105	110	115	119	124	129	134	138
59	89	94	99	104	109	114	119	124	128	133	138	143
60	92	97	102	107	112	118	123	128	133	138	143	148
61	95	100	106	111	116	122	127	132	137	143	148	153
62	98	104	109	115	120	126	131	136	142	147	153	158
63	101	107	113	118	124	130	135	141	146	152	158	163
64	105	110	116	122	128	134	140	145	151	157	163	169
65	108	114	120	126	132	138	144	150	156	162	168	174
66	111	118	124	130	136	142	148	155	161	167	173	179
67	115	121	127	134	140	146	153	159	166	172	178	185
68	118	125	131	138	144	151	158	164	171	177	184	190
69	122	128	135	142	149	155	162	169	176	182	189	196
70	125	132	139	146	153	160	167	174	181	188	195	202
71	129	136	143	150	157	165	172	179	186	193	200	208
72	132	140	147	154	162	169	177	184	191	199	206	213
73	137	144	151	159	166	174	182	189	197	204	212	219
74	141	148	155	163	171	179	186	194	202	210	218	225
75	145	152	160	168	176	184	192	200	208	216	224	232
76	148	156	164	172	180	189	197	205	213	221	230	238

	Very Overweight BMI 30–39									Extremely Overweight
30	31	32	33	34	35	36	37	38	39	40 or more
143	148	153	158	162	167	172	177	181	186	191+
148	153	158	163	168	173	178	183	188	193	198+
153	158	163	168	174	179	184	189	194	199	204+
158	164	169	174	180	185	190	195	201	206	211+
164	169	175	180	186	191	196	202	207	213	218+
169	175	180	186	191	197	203	208	214	220	225+
174	180	186	192	197	204	209	215	221	227	232+
180	186	192	198	204	210	216	222	228	234	240+
186	192	198	204	210	216	223	229	235	241	247+
191	198	204	211	217	223	230	236	242	249	255+
197	203	210	216	223	230	236	243	249	256	262+
203	209	216	223	230	236	243	250	257	263	270+
209	216	223	229	236	243	250	257	264	271	278+
215	222	229	236	243	250	257	265	272	279	286+
221	228	235	242	250	258	265	272	279	287	294+
227	235	242	250	257	265	272	280	288	295	302+
233	241	249	256	264	272	280	287	295	303	311+
240	248	256	264	272	279	287	295	303	311	319+
246	254	263	271	279	287	295	304	312	320	328+

you walk. Think of what it would feel like to carry a 5-pound sack of potatoes wherever you went. Now think of what it would feel like to carry six of those sacks, and the difference to your knees begins to become apparent. When you walk down a flight of stairs, the pressure taken off your knees by a 10-pound weight loss comes to even more—it's akin to being able to let go of 12 sacks of potatoes!

THE CONNECTION BETWEEN DIET AND RHEUMATOID ARTHRITIS

A fishy tale

In general, the saying "you are what you eat" is merely a figure of speech—except when it comes to our consumption of oils, or fats. Different types of oils contain different types of fatty acids. And whatever fatty acids you swallow with the oils you eat are the ones that make their way into the membranes—outer coatings—of every single cell in your body, including the cells in your joints. In other words, the fatty acid makeup of your cell membranes is a direct reflection of the fatty acids you consume.

That fact becomes crucial for those with rheumatoid arthritis. The reason is that fatty acids are precursors of compounds called *prostaglandins,* some of which suppress inflammation and some of which encourage it (see the following table). Of course, someone with rheumatoid arthritis would want to consume oils that lead to the formation of prostaglandins that suppress inflammation, since inflammation in the joint is what causes so much of the pain and stiffness that are the hallmarks of the disease.

So which types of oils contain the fatty acids that best lead to the creation of anti-inflammatory prostaglandins? Fish oils, which come under the category of omega-3 fatty acids. The two most important types of fish oil are eicosapentaenoic acid (EPA) and docosahexaenoic acid (DHA). These oils are found in high concentrations in cold-water fish such as salmon.

Some studies suggesting a benefit from fish oil have looked at supplementation with fish oil capsules, while others have looked at increased consumption of the fish itself.

In one analysis of nine different research projects, fish oil capsules reduced tenderness in three different joints and reduced morning stiffness as

Rating the Oils for Anti-inflammatory or Pro-inflammatory Properties

HIGH ANTI-INFLAMMATORY (RICH IN OMEGA-3 FATTY ACIDS)		
Fish oil		Flaxseed oil
MODERATE ANTI-INFLAMMATORY (MOST ARE RELATIVELY RICH IN OMEGA-3 FATTY ACIDS)		
Canola oil	Soybean oil	Olive oil
Evening primrose oil	Black currant seed oil	Borage oil
PRO-INFLAMMATORY* (RICH IN OMEGA-6 FATTY ACIDS, VIRTUALLY DEVOID OF OMEGA-3s)		
Safflower oil		Sunflower oil
Corn oil		Cottonseed oil

*Minimize use of these oils.

well. The relief was modest, but when the pain is bad enough to keep you from doing the things you like or even being able to rest comfortably, "modest" is pretty good.

As far as eating more fish, a Danish study in which people with rheumatoid arthritis were put on a specialized diet that included an average of 4 ounces of fish every day experienced a significant decrease in morning stiffness, swollen joints, and pain in general after following the regimen for 6 months. They also ended up spending less money on medications to reduce pain and inflammation.

In another study, conducted at the University of Washington, people who ate 2 or more servings of baked or broiled fish every week were 40 percent less likely than those who ate less to end up with arthritis in the future.

An added fish oil benefit

People with rheumatoid arthritis are more prone to heart disease than others. But fish oil appears to have the potential to reduce the risk for heart attacks. It makes blood cells called *platelets* less "sticky" and therefore less prone to form a clot and block the flow of blood to the heart. Fish oil also helps lower blood triglyceride levels, which reduces the risk for heart disease, too.

How to make fish oils work best for you

Fish oil, of course, is just one of many types of oil in the diet. It works against the backdrop of all the other oils you eat. It is those other oils, in fact, that determine how well fish oil can work to ameliorate arthritis symptoms. They can either boost fish oil's capacity to mitigate arthritis pain or hinder it.

Unfortunately, the typical American diet *interferes* with the ability of fish oil to decrease stiffness and pain, which may be why results in studies thus far have been modest. Consider that currently Americans eat only a very tiny proportion of their calories as omega-3 fatty acids. Many more are consumed as omega-6 fatty acids, which, as the table says, promote inflammation. Foods high in omega-6 fatty acids include cottonseed, sunflower, and corn oil, all the processed foods that contain those oils (such as crackers, chips, and other packaged items) and some of the fat in meat. That's a problem on two counts. One is that omega-6 fatty acids can be converted by the body to *arachidonic acid*, which stimulates the formation of prostaglandins that *cause* inflammation. Second, omega-6 fatty acids use the same metabolic pathways in the body as omega-3s; therefore, they compete with each other. Thus, the more omega-6s in the diet, the less chance there is for omega-3s to be metabolized in such a way that they are able to reduce arthritis pain. That's true even for people who take the high doses of omega-3s found in fish oil capsules. The more omega-6s there are that convert to arachidonic acid, the less potential the fish oil has to take up residence in cell membranes and stimulate the production of anti-inflammatory prostaglandins.

We didn't always eat more omega-6s than omega-3s. When humans were still hunter-gatherers and even until the beginning of the 1900s, the ratio of omega-6s to omega-3s was roughly 1:1. That is, we ate the same amounts of the two types of oils. Today, with so many cooking oils rich in omega-6s and so many processed foods manufactured with them, our ratio of omega-6s to omega-3s is more like 11:1. Nutrition scientists in the United States believe we should at least go back to a ratio of 2:1.

So how are we supposed to achieve this ratio? Resort to eating fewer omega-6s and more omega-3s? Exactly. And the good news here is that it does not mean eating tons and tons of fish. That's because omega-3 fatty acids are found not only in fish oil. They're also in a number of plant-derived foods, including canola oil, flaxseed oil, tofu, green leafy vegetables, and nuts. The main omega-3 in these foods is called *alpha-linolenic acid*. Granted, the alpha-linolenic acid in plant foods is not exactly the same as the omega-3s (EPA and DHA) found in fish, which are the best type for ameliorating inflammation and stiffness. But, to some degree, the body can convert them to fish-like omega-3s. More important, these omega-3s don't interfere with the actions of the omega-3s in fish the way omega-6 fatty acids do. Thus, whatever fish you do eat (or fish capsules you take), the omega-3s will be much more effective at alleviating arthritis pain.

A recent study in Australia showed just that. A group of people with rheumatoid arthritis were put on a diet low in omega-6 fatty acids—less than the average intake of 13 grams a day. They were also given capsules of omega-3 fish oils. The result was substantial incorporation of the omega-3 fatty acids into cell membranes—and significant improvements in arthritis symptoms.

In Chapter 4 we will give explicit recommendations for exactly how to increase the proportion of omega-3s in the diet and reduce the proportion of omega-6s. That is, we will show you how to change the "background" diet into which all the other dietary recommendations for ameliorating the pain of arthritis should be incorporated. *Scientists the world over believe that changing the base of the Western diet by shifting the ratio of fatty acids would be a healthful move. That's true not just for people who have rheumatoid arthritis but also for those with osteoarthritis as well as for people who don't have any arthritis at all.*

Don't worry. Your diet won't be weighed down with fish and tofu. But it will contain fewer processed foods along with more green leafy vegetables and other types of produce.

Olive oil—a source of omega-9s

Olive oil is a monounsaturated fat that follows a pathway of metabolism different from those of omega-3s and 6s, as discussed. Relatively few studies have been conducted to see the effects of olive oil on joint pain. So far two of them have shown that it inhibits the inflammatory effects of the omega-6s.

Antioxidants for heading off rheumatoid arthritis pain

As we discussed in Chapter 2, the bodily systems of people with rheumatoid arthritis are on overdrive. Part of the upshot of that is that they are depleted of antioxidants, which are "used up" trying to quench the free radicals involved in causing inflammation. For instance, the level of vitamin C in the joint fluid and blood of people with rheumatoid arthritis is lower than in other people. Research has even suggested that people with low blood levels of antioxidants are more prone than others to *develop* rheumatoid arthritis. A recent study in Finland studied more than 1,400 people and followed them for 20 years. Those who started out with relatively low blood levels of vitamin E and beta-carotene were more than eight times as likely as those with higher blood levels of those antioxidants to end up with the disease as they got older.

In other research conducted in Germany, hospital patients who took 1,200 milligrams of vitamin E each day had the same decrease in morning stiffness, joint tenderness, and joint pain after 3 weeks as those who took nonsteroidal anti-inflammatory drugs (NSAIDs). In another study in England, patients who took 1,200 milligrams of vitamin E daily in addition to their medication suffered less pain than a similar group who took their medications plus a placebo.

B vitamins and rheumatoid arthritis

Studies at Tufts have shown that people with rheumatoid arthritis and, to a lesser extent lupus, have an increased need for vitamins B6 and folate (also a B vitamin). Because of the process of inflammation, it looks like those two nutrients are used up at a faster rate than they are in people without arthritis. Vitamin B6 is found in baked potatoes, bananas, poultry, beef, and fish, while folate is contained in green leafy vegetables, citrus fruits, grain-based foods such as bread and pasta, and brans. There is no evidence that taking more B6 and folate than is contained in a healthful diet or multivitamin is of any use, and it is certainly more expensive.

ALL ARTHRITIS SUFFERERS NEED A SOUND DIET AND EXERCISE PLAN

Of course, since people with rheumatoid arthritis and osteoarthritis both need more antioxidants, there are points of overlap in the dietary recommendations to reduce the pain and disability of the two conditions—a point we made earlier. In fact, despite some wide differences in the dietary research behind the two diseases, there is much about the practical advice on eating that is the same whether you have degenerative or inflammatory arthritis.

It's the same for exercise. Even though osteoarthritis and rheumatoid arthritis work on the body differently, the exercises needed to combat the pain and disability of both conditions are similar. Thus, the basic diet and exercise programs we will be recommending in the following chapters—the cornerstones of our treatment plan—apply to *all* people with arthritis.

As for people afflicted with one of the one hundred or so other kinds of arthritis, there are few or no studies on them because they are each very uncommon. But the mechanisms of joint damage are very similar to those we have described earlier. So it makes sense to approach those more rare forms of arthritis with the same sound diet and exercise program.

The Beat Arthritis Program

CHAPTER 4

Strong Nutrition
for Strong Joints

■

The thing I remember most," says Deborah, "is that it would be very painful to drive a lot of the time—to hold my knee in a bent position. I would wake up in the middle of the night with it. I had to sleep with my legs straight. I would wake up stiff, too."

That was several years ago, around the time Deborah was first diagnosed with osteoarthritis of the knee. Today, the 62-year-old textbook editor doesn't just get out of bed without pain. She also drives without effort. She takes the stairs rather than the elevator to her son's fifth-floor apartment. She completes an annual 20-mile "Walk for Hunger"—all without having to take the ibuprofen that used to make her feel nauseated.

What's different? Her diet, largely. Yet what's ironic is that for all her knee pain has improved, her eating habits haven't changed that dramatically. Yes, there are very definite differences. But Deborah is not fasting or eliminating whole food groups or making other Herculean efforts that for decades have been bandied about—both in books and now on the Internet—as *the* answer to the pain of arthritis. With our help, she has taken simple dietary steps that clinical research suggests may do a lot to quell arthritis pain.

Scientifically sound dietary changes are useful not only for those with *osteo*arthritis. People suffering the stiffness and joint pain of rheumatoid arthritis can mitigate their symptoms, too, by taking the right dietary steps.

The dietary steps for controlling arthritis pain (and perhaps preventing it in the first place) are outlined here, in our Arthritis Diet, complete with a pyramid that you can use as an easy guide for putting together a food plan.

All of our recommendations are based on research findings about the connection between diet and arthritis that we explained in Chapter 3. As you will recall, the underlying keys are eating a healthful diet with the right combination of essential nutrients (vitamins C, D, E, and beta-carotene), consuming the right kinds of unsaturated oils, such as the omega-3 fatty acids found in some fish, vegetables, and vegetable oils, and losing excess weight (if necessary).

THE ARTHRITIS DIET

The Arthritis Food Guide Pyramid is, in many ways, similar to the U.S. Department of Agriculture's Food Guide Pyramid. But there are also several significant differences. As the illustration on the next page shows, grains no longer make up the dietary "base" on which everything else rests. Water does. You could say, in fact, that water keeps the rest of the diet afloat. Fruits and vegetables figure more prominently than grains, too. And among protein-rich foods, fish, beans, and soy foods become more important than beef or poultry.

The whole diet floats on water

You can live without most vitamins and minerals for extended periods of time. But only a few days without water, which is considered an essential nutrient in and of itself, will result in death. Even tissues that don't seem "watery" contain lots of it. Water makes up 75 percent of the muscles, for instance, and more than 20 percent of our bones. (That's right—there's no such thing as being "bone dry.") All together, our bodies are about two-thirds water.

No other substance in the human body is involved in so many functions. Water moisturizes and gives structural support to the joints and other tissues. It carries nutrients and oxygen to the joints as well as to the rest of the body through the blood and lymphatic system. In addition, it plays a crucial role in maintaining body temperature: The heat released when we lose water via evaporation of perspiration helps cool down our bodies.

Water also removes metabolic waste by way of urine, gives "form" to cells, and serves as the medium for thousands of other life-supporting chemical

Arthritis Food Guide Pyramid

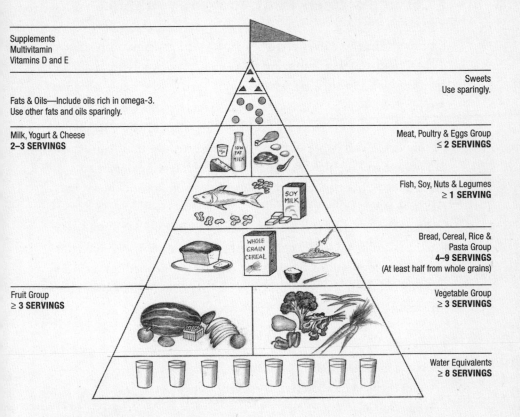

Supplements
Multivitamin
Vitamins D and E

Sweets
Use sparingly.

Fats & Oils—Include oils rich in omega-3.
Use other fats and oils sparingly.

Milk, Yogurt & Cheese
2–3 SERVINGS

Meat, Poultry & Eggs Group
≤ 2 SERVINGS

Fish, Soy, Nuts & Legumes
≥ 1 SERVING

Bread, Cereal, Rice &
Pasta Group
4–9 SERVINGS
(At least half from whole grains)

Fruit Group
≥ 3 SERVINGS

Vegetable Group
≥ 3 SERVINGS

Water Equivalents
≥ 8 SERVINGS

reactions that are constantly going on within us. No wonder water has been referred to as the physiologic river upon which nutrients navigate the pathways of metabolism. As one textbook has put it, nutrients are parched silt and sand at the bottom of a dry riverbed without water. That is, without enough water, all the "right" foods in the world won't be able to properly sustain life.

It might seem as though you don't have to worry about water because when you need more, your body will let you know by making you feel thirsty. But that's not always the case. Thirst is not a perfect mechanism. That's particularly true for people who live in extremely hot climates, people on high-protein diets (which we don't recommend), and the elderly. There is a good deal of evidence that the older we get, the more our capacity to feel thirst

A serving size may not be what you think

Americans these days are often faced with gargantuan portions of food. But what nutrition professionals call a serving is different from what is often perceived—and eaten—as a single serving. A typical deli bagel, for instance, is not 1 serving of bread or even 2 but 5. That's right. A slice of bread is 1 ounce and contains about 80 calories. A deli bagel, on the other hand, weighs on the order of 4–5 ounces and supplies almost 350 calories. A serving of pasta is not the 2–3 cups of spaghetti you might get at an Italian eatery but, rather, ½ cup.

That doesn't mean you should never eat more than ½ cup of pasta at a time. But if you have 2 cups' worth, you're eating 4 servings from the grains group out of the 4–9 servings recommended for a single day. Following are the recommended serving sizes of items from the various food groups.

Fruits
    1 medium apple, banana, or orange
    ½ cup chopped (raw, cooked, or canned) fruit
    ¾ cup fruit juice

Vegetables
    1 cup raw leafy greens (lettuce, spinach, etc.)
    ½ cup other vegetables, cooked
    ¾ cup vegetable juice

Grains
    1-ounce slice of bread
    1 ounce ready-to-eat cereal
    ½ cup cooked cereal, rice, or pasta
    ¼ large bagel

Fish, soy foods, eggs, dried beans, and nuts
   3 ounces fish
   ½ cup soybeans or tofu
   ½ cup cook dried beans
   1 egg, 2 tablespoons peanut butter, or ½–1 ounce nuts

Milk, yogurt, and cheese
   1 cup milk or yogurt
   1½ ounces hard cheese

Meat, poultry, and pork
   3 ounces cooked lean beef, poultry, or pork

when necessary becomes blunted. Some of the medicines used to treat arthritis can also affect thirst.

Because the thirst sensation does not always kick in when it should, **we advise everyone to drink at least 8 cups of fluid a day, preferably water.** Juices and (noncaffeinated) soda pop will take care of your fluid needs, but at great caloric expense. And caffeinated beverages, including coffee, tea, and many sodas, are diuretics, which means they tend to draw water from you. Granted, you'll take in more water from a cup of coffee than it will cause you to excrete in the urine, but it still causes greater fluid losses than water itself. So does alcohol, which also has a diuretic effect.

The produce bin takes on new prominence

It's critical to eat 3 or more servings of fruit daily and 3 or more servings of vegetables. They are the only food groups that contain substantial amounts of vitamin C, beta-carotene, and folate—nutrients that people with osteoarthritis and rheumatoid arthritis need more of than others, according to research findings to date.

How much vitamin C should you be aiming for each day? While the Daily Value for the general population is 75 milligrams, we suggest 200 milligrams.

In cases of osteoarthritis, vitamin C at this level appears to help reduce pain. And those with rheumatoid arthritis apparently "use up" much more vitamin C than others, requiring a greater supply.

Fortunately, if you're eating a daily minimum of three fruits and three vegetables for a total of at least 6 servings of produce (which will also help with any weight-control effort), it's fairly easy to reach the 200-milligram mark. You need never rely solely on a supplement. Check out the various combinations in the box that follows. As you browse, keep in mind that they're only suggestions. The important thing is to go for a wide variety of vegetables and fruits. As long as you eat plenty of them and vary your sources rather than eat the same ones day after day, you're sure to get all the vitamin C you need—especially if you don't always stick to 6 servings. Remember, that's a minimum, not a limit.

The beta-carotene connection

For beta-carotene, there is no Daily Value or recommended allowance. However, as you will recall, people with osteoarthritis who consumed at least 9,000 IU daily were at a reduced risk for disease progression compared to those who ate fewer than 5,000 IU. Taking in at least 9,000 IU of beta-carotene daily is also important for people with rheumatoid arthritis. Certainly, it appears to be a good thing for *avoiding* it, since research has indicated that those with low blood levels of beta-carotene are much more likely to develop the disease.

The best sources of beta-carotene are listed in the box on p. 60. Whatever you do, DON'T take single-nutrient beta-carotene pills. It's fine if there's up to 5,000 IU of beta-carotene in a multivitamin supplement that you might be taking, but large doses of beta-carotene in pill form have been found to be harmful for some groups of people, including smokers, former smokers, and workers exposed to asbestos.

Note that some of the sources of both vitamin C and beta-carotene are green leafy vegetables, such as broccoli, Brussels sprouts, spinach, kale, and collard greens. Green leafy vegetables (collards and kale, in particular) also contain some of the omega-3 fatty acids that lead to the formation in cell membranes of prostaglandins that work to inhibit inflammation. The

Three diet combinations that provide 200+ milligrams of vitamin C

Combination 1:

6 ounces orange juice	73
½ cup spaghetti sauce	18
1 kiwifruit	75
1 banana	10
½ cup cooked broccoli	37
1 medium baked potato	20
Total:	233 mg

Combination 2:

1 cup strawberries	85
1 cup cantaloupe pieces	68
1 medium peach	6
½ cup cooked cauliflower	13
1 baked sweet potato with skin	28
8 frozen asparagus spears	30
Total:	230 mg

Combination 3:

½ grapefruit	39
1 orange	75
½ cup chopped green pepper	45
6 ounces vegetable juice cocktail	50
½ cup cooked Brussels sprouts	18
1 cup honeydew pieces	42
Total:	269 mg

The best sources of beta-carotene, in International Units (IU)

Shoot for at least 9,000 IU of beta-carotene a day from food.

½ cup canned pumpkin	26,908
1 baked sweet potato	24,877
1 medium carrot	20,253
1 medium mango	8,061
½ cup frozen spinach, boiled	7,395
1 cup cantaloupe pieces	5,158
½ cup chopped frozen collard greens, boiled	5,084
½ cup chopped frozen kale, boiled	4,810
½ cup mashed frozen butternut squash	4,007
3 medium apricots	2,769
6 ounces vegetable juice cocktail	2,129
½ cup frozen broccoli, boiled	1,741
5 dried peach halves	1,406
1 medium nectarine	1,001
1 medium papaya	863
1 medium tangerine	773

green vegetable *highest* in omega-3 fatty acids is purslane, a staple in the Mediterranean diet that's not commonly eaten in North America but is grown in all fifty states. Ask for it at your local grocer—an increase in the demand for it may make it more readily available.

Going with grains

There has been a great deal of confusion about grains, or starchy foods, over the last several years. Proponents of fad diets have said they do everything from leave you hungry to make you fat. It's not true. Many traditional cultures, from those in Europe to those in the Far East, have depended on grains as an integral part of their diets for centuries and have been none the worse for it. Indeed, the traditional Japanese and Chinese diets are based largely on grains in the form of rice, and people in China and Japan have historically been quite lean and free of the diseases that plague many in the United States and other Western nations: heart disease, diabetes, and several types of cancer.

Having said this, we do feel that most people eat too *many* grains (especially refined grains) and that has probably contributed to the increased weight gain that Americans have experienced over the past few decades. We recommend that you consume 4–9 servings a day of grains, a couple of servings less than the U.S. Department of Agriculture recommends. Remember that a single serving of pasta is just ½ cup—not much more than fits into an ice cream scooper.

Note that you should not be making white bread or pasta, both refined grains, the mainstays of your grain choices. We recommend that you choose *whole* grains such as whole-grain breads and breakfast cereals, oatmeal and brown rice, along with perhaps some lesser-utilized whole grains such as bulgur, barley, and wheat berries. The reason is twofold. First, whole grains, as opposed to refined grains like those in white bread, most bagels, spaghetti, and white rice, contain fiber, which Americans do not get enough of. Currently, we consume about 10–15 grams of fiber daily, when the goal is 25 grams.

Second, whole grains are much richer in certain key nutrients than refined, or processed, grains. When grains are processed, B vitamins, vitamin E, zinc, iron, selenium, magnesium, and other minerals are lost. Granted, some of those nutrients are added back—"enriched" refined grains contain B vitamins and iron, for instance. But most nutrients that were there to begin with are left out.

A new spin on protein

Protein is an essential nutrient. The protein in our diet supplies *amino acids*—the building blocks for structural components in the body (muscles, cartilage, and bone), hormones, and many of the molecules that comprise the immune system as well as other biological systems in the body. Protein can also be used as a source of energy. It's easy to see why adequate intake is essential. But "adequate" is not the same for everyone.

Balance your grains

Agood rule of thumb is to make at least half of your daily grain choices whole grain. If you eat, say, 5 servings of grains a day, you might want to start with a breakfast of whole-grain cereal (oats are one whole-grain option, but there are many others) and then have a sandwich made with two slices of whole-grain bread for lunch. (Check ingredients lists to make sure the first ingredient on the label says *whole* grain or 100 percent *whole* wheat, not simply "multigrain" or "unbromated" or "unbleached" flour.) Then, at dinner, you could have ½ cup of rice or pasta. A couple of cookies or a thin slice of cake for dessert also contains about one serving of refined grains. Of course, the more whole grains that make up the daily starch intake, the better.

The protein requirement is higher for people with rheumatoid arthritis than for others because they have a condition associated with the disease called *rheumatoid cachexia* (see Chapter 3). As a result, they experience increased protein breakdown in the body, which leads to the loss of muscle.

Aside from being important in itself, protein contributes largely to the types of fats we consume because foods high in protein often come coupled with various types of fat. And, as we explained in Chapter 3, it's very important for the diet to have the proper ratios of various fatty acids in order to reduce the potential for inflammation at the joint. Indeed, it's very important for *everyone* to have the proper fatty acid ratios for good health in general. The aim is to consume more omega-3 fatty acids and fewer omega-6 fatty acids and saturated fats.

Health experts from Canada to Denmark to Japan have spelled out recommendations for doing just that. The World Health Organization, too, believes people should aim for more omega-3s. At present, we average only about 1 gram of omega-3s daily, when we should be taking in more on the order of 3 grams: 0.7 grams from fish and 2.3 grams from other foods. The protein recommendations here will assure a significantly higher omega-3 intake and a better omega-3:omega-6 ratio and thus help to reduce inflammation.

One of those recommendations is to eat more cold-water fish, the most important protein in your diet if you have arthritis (see the table on the following page for a list of cold-water fish). Cold-water species are the only rich source of the two most effective omega-3 fatty acids (EPA and DHA) that are so important in fighting the inflammatory process of arthritis. They are also low in the pro-inflammatory omega-6 oils. Meats (beef, chicken, and pork), on the other hand, have virtually no EPA or DHA and very little other omega-3s, but they have significantly more omega-6s, -9s, and saturated fat.

Aside from adding fish to the diet, choosing more vegetable proteins—tofu, beans, nuts, and seeds—will also boost your intake of omega-3s. And, like fish, they will automatically limit your consumption of undesirable fats when they replace meat.

It's for these reasons that vegetable proteins, along with fish, are closer to the foundation of the food pyramid than meat. We're not saying you should never eat beef, chicken, and pork. But they should assume a smaller role in your diet, as these other protein sources are included in more of your meals. See the following table for a list of various foods and their contribution to the omega-3s in the diet.

Eating 4 servings of fish a week should guarantee the recommended consumption level of the two omega-3 fatty acids found only in fish. You only need to eat fish several times a week rather than every day because many types of fish contain significantly more than 0.7 grams of omega-3 in a serving. You can average out your intake over the course of a week.

For the other omega-3s, if you choose the right oils (which we will talk about more in the section on fat) and substitute some vegetable protein for meat dishes and add some nuts here and there, you will easily meet the 2.3-gram recommendation. Making these choices will also automatically cut down on the saturated and other fatty acids in foods like meat and poultry, which have the potential to compete with omega-3s in the body and thereby *contribute* to inflammation at the joint.

We recognize that what we're recommending here may be a fairly big change for many. After all, some people hardly ever eat fish. And relatively few people regularly include nuts or seeds in their diets—or tofu, for that matter. If making this wholesale dietary shift seems too overwhelming, don't

OMEGA-3 CONTENT OF VARIOUS FOODS

Food	Omega-3s (linolenic acid), in grams	Omega-3s (EPA and DHA), in grams
Fish (3 ozs.)		
Bluefish	0	0.84
Halibut	0.07	0.40
Mackerel (Atlantic)	0.10	1.00
Salmon (Coho, farmed)	0.07	1.09
Salmon (Coho, wild)	0.05	0.90
Salmon (Sockeye with bones, canned)	0.08	0.98
Sardines (oil drained with bones, canned)	0.42	0.83
Swordfish	0.20	0.70
Trout (rainbow wild)	0.16	0.84
Tuna (fresh bluefin)	0	1.28
Tuna (canned, white)	0	0.73
Nuts and seeds (1 oz.)		
Butternuts	2.47	0
Pecans	0.28	0
Soy nuts	0.48	0
Walnuts (black)	0.94	0
Walnuts (English)	2.57	0
Flaxseeds	4.35	0
Vegetable proteins (½ cup)		
Black beans	0.09	0
Kidney beans	0.14	0
Pinto beans	0.20	0

Vegetable proteins (½ cup) *continued*		
Soybeans (green, cooked)	0.32	0
Tofu (raw firm)	0.40	0
Vegetables (½ cup)		
Collards (cooked)	0.09	0
Kale (cooked)	0.07	0
Spinach (cooked)	0.08	0
Oils (1 tablespoon)		
Canola	1.30	0
Flaxseed	8.00	0
Soybean	0.93	0
Walnut	1.40	0

try it all at once. Even going from no fish meals a week to just one or two is a great improvement. Likewise, try sprinkling a small handful of nuts or seeds on your salad just a couple of times a week. (You might even find that you like the taste and texture!) Any inroads you can make to increase the proportion of omega-3s in your diet while cutting down on calories from other sources will help your joints.

Note: The research on fish oil capsules discussed in Chapter 3 used much higher doses than what we are recommending here. The requirements we have just spoken about are for the background diet for *everyone*. We will discuss supplementing on top of this in the supplement section later in this chapter.

Dairy dos and don'ts

Two to 3 servings of dairy foods a day are important to the health of your bones, which are so integrally involved in joint function. If some of your dairy choices are milk, so much the better. All milk in this country is fortified with vitamin D, which research has shown to be crucial for joint health. One cup of milk has 100 IU of vitamin D.

What about mercury in fish?

Mercury is a naturally occurring mineral that is released from the earth's crust and oceans into the atmosphere. It is also released into the air via various types of pollution, such as when fossil fuels like coal are burned. This combination of events causes mercury to accumulate in streams, lakes, and oceans. When mercury combines with certain bacteria in water, a chemical reaction occurs, converting mercury to methyl mercury, which can be toxic.

Fish and other aquatic life absorb the methyl mercury as it passes over their gills and when they eat. Larger predator fish are vulnerable to higher methyl mercury levels because they are getting methyl mercury from two sources: from absorption through their gills and from muscle tissue of the smaller fish they consume for food.

In March 2001, the FDA issued a warning about toxic levels of methyl mercury (greater than 1 part per million) in certain large predatory fish. The fish FDA scientists are concerned about include *shark, swordfish, king mackerel, and tilefish.*

For healthy adults: Consume no more than 14 ounces per week of the types of fish listed above. All other fish are fine.

For children, women of childbearing age, and especially pregnant women: The official recommendation is to avoid these types of fish altogether. This is because high levels of methyl mercury can damage a developing nervous system. For other varieties of fish and seafood—salmon, cod, canned tuna, clams, scallops, and others—up to 12 ounces per week are fine.

For specific questions about methyl mercury and fish and seafood as well as current recommendations, go to www.fda.gov or call the FDA at 1-888-SAFEFOOD.

Try to make as many of your dairy choices as possible low-fat or non-fat. Many people are not aware that full-fat dairy foods, cheeses in particular, often contain as much saturated fat (which can lead to clogged arteries) as a well-marbled cut of beef. If full-fat dairy is the only way to go for you taste-wise, be cognizant of the amount you eat. A single serving of cheese amounts to only 1½ ounces—the size of just two dominoes.

If dairy is not for you, there are options that can help fill the void. Soy milk is widely available today, and many brands come fortified with vitamin D and calcium (check labels). Other fortified soy products, such as tofu enriched with calcium, can also help take the place of dairy foods, although they don't tend to contain quite as much calcium and are often devoid of vitamin D.

The omega-3 contribution of fats/oils

Protein-containing foods are not the only possibilities for shifting the ratio of fatty acids in the diet so that it includes a higher proportion of omega-3s and less of other fatty acids. Fats, or cooking (vegetable) oils themselves, play a significant role. Currently, the cooking oils Americans most commonly eat are high in omega-6 fatty acids. These are polyunsaturated fatty acids in items like corn, safflower, and cottonseed oil, which we currently eat ten times as much of as oils that contain omega-3s. It would be better for health if we ate only two to three times as much omega-6s as omega-3s. One way to do that is to make a shift in cooking oils: less corn, safflower, and cottonseed oil and more canola and soybean oil. Although they still contain omega-6s, they have higher quantities of omega-3s than corn, safflower, and cottonseed oils.

Many people have already made the switch to canola oil in their pantries. But a large portion of the corn and cottonseed oil we eat comes not from the oil in the cupboard that we cook with but from processed foods—everything from many kinds of crackers to rice and stuffing mixes to prepared frozen and boxed foods and many dessert items. Thus, the fewer processed foods you buy and the more unrefined whole foods you eat—whole-grain breads and cereals, vegetables, fruits, nuts, seeds, beans, and small portions of meat and dairy foods—the higher your ratio of omega-3 fatty acids to omega-6s will automatically be. (See the table on page 65 for a list of the omega-3s in cooking oils.)

Another oil to use in your diet is olive oil, which is high in the mono-unsaturated omega-9 fatty acids. There is less research on this oil regarding

Flaxseed oil to the rescue

One of the best oils you can add to your diet is flaxseed—among the richest vegetable sources of omega-3 fatty acids. Flaxseed oil can be found in many mainstream grocery stores that have a "natural foods" section and in any health-food store. The oil is unrefined, comes in small quantities, and is kept refrigerated in a dark bottle. It is treated this way because the fatty acids contained in it are easily damaged when exposed to light, heat, and air. Flaxseed oil should not be heated (used in cooking); the fatty acids will be damaged and therefore not have the same beneficial properties. Use it on salads, mixed into yogurt, or as a dip for bread with some herbs added.

arthritis, but it, too, has been shown to decrease inflammation. In addition, substituting olive oil for corn and safflower oil, where possible, will help replace some of the omega-6s in the diet.

Sweets and snack foods

We won't belabor the point. Candies, cookies, cakes, pies, ice cream, pudding, soda pop, corn chips, potato chips, and beer nuts are all delicious. And they should all be *occasional* additions to your eating plan, not dietary mainstays. According to government surveys, 25 percent of our calories currently come from such foods. That number should be closer to 5 percent.

Supplements as an insurance policy

We know you are going to make the best effort to follow the Arthritis Diet, but just to play it safe we recommend that you take a multivitamin (with iron for women of childbearing years and without iron for men and post-menopausal women) to make sure your nutritional bases are *always* covered. There are also some specific vitamins that appear to help arthritis symptoms, and they differ depending on whether you have osteoarthritis or rheumatoid arthritis.

Vitamin D: a supplement to consider if you have osteoarthritis

As we said in Chapter 3, research has suggested that 400 IU of vitamin D each day seems to protect people from disease progression—not to mention from the development of osteoporosis. It also happens to be the Recommended Daily Allowance for people 51–70 years old. (Until age 50, the recommended allowance is 200 IU; above age 70, it's 600 IU.) Thus, we believe that everyone through age 70 who has osteoarthritis should be shooting for 400 IU a day. Once you turn 71, increase daily intake to 600 IU.

The problem here is that it's hard to take in 400 IU of vitamin D from food alone. Milk is the greatest dietary source of that nutrient (which is not a natural component—milk is fortified), and it contains only 100 IU per cup. And few people drink 4 cups of milk a day. Fatty fish such as salmon and mackerel have a little vitamin D, too, but not very much. And breakfast cereal, if it's fortified with vitamin D, contains only about 40 IU per serving.

Compounding the problem is that although we synthesize vitamin D in our skin when it is exposed to sunlight (hence its moniker, "the sunshine vitamin"), the skin becomes much less efficient at making vitamin D as we age. In addition, the kidneys become less capable of converting the nutrient to a form that is usable by the body. Worse still, for people who live above the 40-degree-latitude line (think of a line stretching from Philadelphia through Denver to northern California), the sunlight isn't strong enough to make any vitamin D in January and February. If you live at or north of the 42-degree line (think of a line stretching from Boston through Chicago to somewhere near the California/Oregon border), your skin doesn't make any vitamin D from early November through early March.

For all these reasons, we recommend that you get at least some of your vitamin D from a supplement. Many multivitamins contain 200 IU, so if you drink 2 cups of milk per day (in coffee, with cereal, or as part of soups, puddings, and casseroles) and take a multivitamin that contains vitamin D, you'll be fine. If you don't drink any milk whatsoever (although we recommend that you do, not just for the vitamin D but also for protein, calcium, riboflavin, and other nutrients), take a multivitamin that contains 400 IU of vitamin D until you reach age 71, at which point you should be getting 600 IU daily. Some multivitamin supplements made specifically for people older than 50 contain 400–600 IU of the nutrient.

During the warm-weather months, try to get 10–15 minutes of sun each day on your arms or legs without sunscreen, which blocks vitamin D synthesis (always cover your face with sunscreen). Or, if you're very fair, take 10–15 minutes in the sun twice a week with a sunscreen that has a Sun Protection Factor (SPF) of 6–8. You won't burn or predispose yourself to skin cancer if you limit your sun exposure to the amount we recommend.

Whatever you do, don't take more than 1,000 IU of vitamin D daily in supplemental form. The official upper limit is 2,000 IU, but there have been reports of toxicity from 1,000 IU. At that level, you can begin to *hasten* bone loss and have other complications.

Fish oil: a supplement to consider if you have rheumatoid arthritis

Everyone should be following the Arthritis Diet to increase the proportion of omega-3 fatty acids in their diets. But a significant amount of research suggests that people with rheumatoid arthritis have to consume much more of the omega-3s in fish (EPA and DHA) to reduce pain and stiffness. Whereas the Arthritis Diet contains a little less than 1 gram combined of EPA and DHA, some studies in which symptoms of arthritis improved used supplements at higher doses—3–6 grams. Even if you ate the very best fish sources, to get to those high amounts you'd be eating much more fish than anyone could reasonably be expected to include in the diet—a minimum of 3 servings of salmon every single day, for instance, or at least 5 servings of canned tuna.

For that reason, we suggest that people who want to try fish oil specifically for reducing arthritis pain use fish oil capsules. We recommend that you first discuss it with your doctor, and make sure there are no issues, such as other health problems or medications that could conflict with the fish oil. If you decide to go ahead, supplement with between 3 and 6 grams a day. Try the fish oil capsules for 12 weeks straight, even if you don't feel any differences along the way. It generally takes at least 12 weeks before people start to observe improvements. If at around 12 weeks you notice less pain and tenderness, try the capsules for another 6–12 weeks. The improvements appear to increase if the treatment lasts that long. If you don't notice an effect by then, stop the capsules.

Be aware that going on a fish oil regimen is not something that everybody will find easy. Many capsules contain only about 300 milligrams of omega-3 fatty acids, meaning that it takes ten capsules just to reach 3 grams (although 800 milligrams are now also available). Furthermore, many who take them end up with fishy-smelling belches. Also, fish oil can increase the risk for bleeding, say, in the case of an accident or surgery, so a doctor should be monitoring you.

Fish oil pills are not a substitute for the Arthritis Diet. As we said earlier, the beneficial effects of fish oil have been modest. But we suspect that's because people are following diets that are too low in omega-3s—and too high in other fatty acids—to begin with. On the Arthritis Diet, the ratio of fatty acids is better, which has the effect of giving the fatty acids in the pills a better chance of quelling arthritis pain. It's a diet that serves as the best "background" against which the supplements can do their work.

Indeed, for some people, omega-3 supplements may be able to replace anti-inflammatory drugs like NSAIDs, at least to some degree (and as long as your doctor says it's okay). That could mean coping with fewer of those drugs' side effects, including stomach discomfort, gastrointestinal bleeding, and ulcers.

Caution: Do *not* take large amounts of cod liver oil or any other fish oil preparations that have not been stripped of vitamins A and D. In large doses, those two nutrients can be toxic to the liver.

Calcium: a supplement to consider if you have rheumatoid arthritis

Many people, particularly women, fall woefully short of their calcium needs and would benefit from taking a calcium supplement. Consider that women through age 50 are advised to consume 1,000 milligrams of calcium daily and that women 51 and older should shoot for 1,200 milligrams, yet many women *of all ages* take in more on the order of 600 milligrams. The shortfall becomes particularly problematic for anyone with rheumatoid arthritis because people with that form of the disease have a very accelerated rate of osteoporosis—calcium depletion from the skeleton that leads to bone thinning and an increased risk for fractures. These women's calcium losses become even greater if they take prednisone. That's why we recommend that *all* people with rheumatoid and other inflammatory forms of arthritis take 800–1,200 milligrams daily of calcium supplements, preferably calcium citrate.

Vitamin E: a supplement to consider for osteoarthritis or rheumatoid arthritis
We have told you that studies on both osteoarthritis and rheumatoid arthritis have suggested that supplements of vitamin E can reduce pain and stiffness. But while the evidence sounds promising, it is still scant. Therefore, we cannot definitively recommend that you take supplemental doses of vitamin E to reduce arthritis discomfort. However, if you want to try it, we think it *may* be helpful and, at the very least, won't be harmful.

The German study on osteoarthritis (discussed in Chapter 3) lasted no longer than 6 weeks, so if you don't feel better with vitamin E supplements after a couple of months, you're probably not going to. Make sure to stick to 400 milligrams a day. Very high doses could increase the risk for bleeding.

With rheumatoid arthritis, it gets a little complicated. The studies showing that vitamin E reduces stiffness, joint tenderness, and pain were conducted with 1,200 milligrams of vitamin E per patient each day. However, the Institute of Medicine says the safe upper limit for vitamin E is 1,000 milligrams a day because of the bleeding potential with higher amounts. For that reason, we suggest you discuss dosage with your doctor. Certainly, if you are taking an anticoagulant drug such as Coumadin (warfarin) or have an operation scheduled where the risks of losing blood are magnified, your physician will probably recommend that you stick to 1,000 milligrams a day—at most—and not reach the 1,200-milligram mark. Whatever dose of vitamin E you and your physician may decide on, try it for only a couple of months to see whether it's benefiting you. If you don't see any effect within 8 weeks or so, there's very little chance that continuing will do any good.

LOSING EXCESS WEIGHT

Following the Arthritis Diet can go a long way to help people with osteoarthritis shed some of the extra weight that exacerbates their pain. After all, the processed foods that should become a smaller part of the daily eating

Are you getting enough vitamin E from food?

It certainly pays to eat enough vitamin E as part of your diet, particularly if you have osteoarthritis. As you will recall, people with knee arthritis in the Framingham study did much better if they consumed at least 6–11 milligrams of vitamin E daily. Higher amounts of vitamin E are also needed when you increase the amount of fish oil in your diet. Fish oil is susceptible to breakdown, and vitamin E can stabilize the oil.

Estimates of the amount of vitamin E Americans consume are spotty, although some surveys suggest we're taking in an average of 9–10 milligrams daily. The Recommended Dietary Allowance is 15 milligrams. Here are some of the best sources.

	Milligrams of vitamin E
1 ounce sunflower seeds	14
1 ounce hazelnuts or almonds	7
1 tablespoon sunflower oil	7
1 tablespoon safflower oil	6
¼ cup toasted wheat germ	5
2 tablespoons almond butter	6
2 tablespoons peanut butter	3
1 papaya	3
1 mango	2
⅓ cup granola	2
3 ounces cooked flounder or sole	2
1 cup condensed tomato soup prepared with water	2

plan tend to be high in calories, while fruits, vegetables, and whole grains help people feel full on fewer calories, and fish tends to have fewer calories per serving than meat. That is, switching to the Arthritis Diet will automatically give a head start to those wanting to shed pounds to help reduce the symptoms of their disease. In many cases, it might be all an overweight person needs, even if it doesn't get him or her model-slim.

Small weight loss, big rewards

As we said in Chapter 3, research has shown that a weight loss of just 2 units of BMI (see the chart on pages 42–43)—which for most people amounts to about 11 pounds—can decrease the pain and stiffness of osteoarthritis by up to 50 percent! Gaining that much weight can increase the severity of symptoms by a similar amount. Another way of looking at it is that even maintaining weight, rather than gaining, can do a lot to prevent unnecessary pain.

So forget about "ideal" weight here in terms of easing—or preventing—pain and stiffness. (The government forgot about it years ago. They now talk in terms of "healthy" weight.) Don't worry about losing dozens of pounds. If you're overweight, we want you to focus on taking the small step of just a 5- to 10-pound weight loss. It can have a dramatic effect. If you want to try to lose more weight after your initial weight loss, you can think about that afterward.

Take your time. You didn't gain 5–10 pounds in a week. There's no reason to try to lose it that fast. Even taking 6 months to lose 10 pounds is perfectly reasonable. That's about how long Deborah took. And she didn't even lose 10 pounds. She lost only about 5. But it was enough to make a difference. After all, a 5-pound loss is akin to taking 15 pounds of pressure off your knee— 30 pounds if you're walking down a flight of stairs.

How to do it? We don't recommend the extremely high-protein plans currently fashionable. There's no scientific evidence that people who follow them keep off the weight over the long term. In addition, they can be dangerous for people who have kidney or liver problems.

Rather, we propose sticking carefully to the Arthritis Diet—plenty of vegetables and fruits (6–9 servings a day, with at least as many vegetables as fruits); reasonable amounts of whole grains (and few refined grains); smallish portions of fish, beans, soy, nuts, seeds, and eggs (and fewer portions of beef, pork, and poultry); 2–3 daily servings of low- and non-fat dairy foods; and little in the way of sweets and "munchies" like potato chips. Researchers at the University of Pittsburgh and the University of Colorado who are keeping a National Weight Control Registry of thousands of people who have lost at least 30 pounds—and kept off the weight for at least 1 year—have found evidence through surveys suggesting that's the way successful weight losers' diets shape up.

More than 90 percent of them also exercise on a regular basis to *keep off* the weight. Both aerobic activities such as brisk walking and the strength training described in Chapter 5 burn calories and help maintain weight loss.

THE ARTHRITIS DIET: SAMPLE MENUS

Below are three menus to feed your joints: one vegetarian, one with fish and meat, and one with fish but no meat. They provide the recommended 6 or more servings of fruits and vegetables and the proper amounts of omega-3 fatty acids. Each menu contains 1,900–2,000 calories, the amount an active woman may require. Active men may need more calories. In addition, because many people are trying to lose weight, we have included adaptations to

Strong Women Stay Slim to help you jump-start your weight-loss effort

Strong Women Stay Slim (whose advice applies equally well to men), written by Miriam Nelson and Sarah Wernick, offers a variety of eating plans in the 1,200-, 1,600-, and 2,000-calorie ranges designed to help you lose weight sensibly and effectively. There are plans for sweets eaters, vegetarians, and the "I'm always hungry" crowd (which stretches out the day's calories among foods that are not calorically dense so the weight loser can keep eating). The book also includes fifty mouth-watering recipes created by award-winning chef Steven Raichlen, who has penned more than a dozen cookbooks.

reduce each menu to 1,600 calories. The adaptations for 1,600 calories still provide adequate fruit and vegetable intake and omega-3 fatty acids. Use the menus as a starting point or for ideas to customize menus to suit your own food preferences.

As the menus illustrate, following them does not call for Draconian switches in your eating habits or for punishing restraint. Deborah increased her intake of such nutrients as vitamin C and beta-carotene simply by making gradual changes in her diet that she says "didn't feel intrusive or corrective." For instance, she recounts, "I really like fruits. So I eat a lot of them—and a lot of vegetables. I love sweets, but I haven't been having much of them." In other words, the better you feel, the less you want to continue your old way of eating, even if you liked the way it tasted. You just don't want to put yourself through the pain that your old way of eating contributed to.

One way Deborah maintains a better diet is by being more *mindful* of what she puts in her mouth. Before, when she was feeling stressed, she would go to Burger King and numb herself with a fried chicken sandwich. Now, she says, "I'll wait till I get home." And she thinks carefully about what to prepare for herself so that it will be in line with the healthful diet she believes is helping to keep her pain in check. "It's a process of learning how to cook," she comments. "It makes you aware not only of ingredients but also of portion sizes."

Vegetarian Menu

Meal	Menu	Omega-3 Fatty Acids	Calories
Breakfast	1 cup shredded wheat		152
	1 cup skim milk		90
	1 banana		109
	¾ cup orange juice		84
	1 tablespoon flaxseeds on cereal	2.2 g	59
Lunch	1 whole-wheat pita pocket		170
	½ cup hummus		210
	½ tomato		13
	1 cup lettuce		9
	8 baby carrots		30
	2 fig bars		111
Dinner	Tofu and greens stir-fry		
	½ cup tofu	0.4 g	130
	¾ cup Swiss chard		26
	1 cup brown rice *or* white rice		
	or mixed		216
	Sauce		234
	1 tablespoon Canola oil	1.3 g	
	1 tablespoon rice vinegar		
	2 tablespoons cooking sherry		
	¾ tablespoon brown sugar		
	¼ oz. ginger slices		
	¾ tablespoon lime juice		
	½ tablespoon cilantro		
	2 tablespoons soy sauce		

Meal	Menu	Omega-3 Fatty Acids	Calories
Snacks	1 cup non-fat yogurt sweetened with ¼ cup strawberries		148
	½ oz. English walnuts, raw or roasted	1.3 g	93
	1 large apple		125
Total omega-3 fats = 5.2 g.			

Adaptations to the menu for 1,600 calories:

Reduce shredded wheat cereal to ¾ cup.

Reduce skim milk to ½ cup.

Omit fig bars, walnuts, and apples.

Fish and Meat Menu

Meal	Menu	Omega-3 Fatty Acids	Calories
Breakfast	Smoothie		
	1 cup low-fat plain yogurt		155
	½ cup orange juice		56
	½ cup strawberries		22
	¼ cup blueberries		20
	1 banana		109
	1 tablespoon flaxseed oil	8 g	130
Lunch	Turkey sandwich		
	2 slices whole-wheat bread		138
	4 oz. sliced turkey breast		193
	1 oz. cheese		114
	½ tomato		13
	3 leaves lettuce		5
	1 tablespoon mustard		15
	3 oatmeal raisin cookies		196
Dinner	Broiled salmon		
	5 oz. salmon	1.92 g (1.8 is EPA and DHA)	330
	½ tomato		
	Slice of onion		
	Wedge of lemon		
	Dill		
	1 cup couscous		176
	1 cup sautéed spinach with garlic and 1 tsp. olive oil	0.15 g	82

Meal	Menu	Omega-3 Fatty Acids	Calories
Snacks	1 cup frozen yogurt 8 baby carrots		229 30
Total omega-3 fats = 10 g.			

Adaptations to the menu for 1,600 calories:

Reduce turkey breast slices to 3 oz.

Omit cookies and cheese on sandwich.

Reduce frozen yogurt to ½ cup.

Fish Menu

Meal	Menu	Omega-3 Fatty Acids	Calories
Breakfast	1 cup oatmeal		145
	2 tablespoons raisins		54
	1 small apple		81
	1 cup milk (1% fat)		102
	¾ cup orange juice		83
Lunch	Veggie burrito		
	8-inch tortilla		159
	¼ cup salsa		12
	½ cup black beans		114
	½ cup white rice		103
	¼ cup zucchini and yellow squash		9
	⅛ cup eggplant		4
	1 oz. cheese		114
Dinner	Tuna and pasta		
	5 oz. tuna	0.80 g (0.73 is EPA and DHA)	164
	Sauce		58
	½ cup canned tomatoes		
	¼ tablespoon olive oil		
	Garlic, parsley		
	1½ cups macaroni (½ whole-wheat, ½ white)		278
	1 cup steamed broccoli and cauliflower		44

Meal	Menu	Omega-3 Fatty Acids	Calories
Dinner *(cont.)*	Salad		
	1½ cups green leafy lettuce, carrots, and peppers		33
	2½ tablespoon dressing: olive oil, vinegar, and mustard		254
	2 tablespoons Parmesan cheese		57
Add-ins *(choose one)*	Add flaxseed oil to your oatmeal *or* sprinkle flax seeds *or* roasted walnuts on your salad.		
	½ tablespoon flaxseed oil	4 g	65
	1 tablespoon flaxseeds	2.2 g	59
	½ oz. English walnuts	1.3 g	93

Total omega-3 fats = 4.8 total g (using the flaxseed oil add-in; lower if you add in flaxseeds or walnuts).

Adaptations to the menu for 1,600 calories:

Reduce oatmeal to ½ cup.

Reduce 1% milk to ½ cup.

Reduce rice to ¼ cup.

Reduce pasta to ¾ cup.

Reduce tuna to 4 oz.

Use 1 tablespoon flaxseeds as your add-in.

CHAPTER 5

The Beat Arthritis Exercise Program

◼

Six weeks after my youngest son was born, it hit me," says Liz, mother of three boys. "I couldn't lift him out of his crib at night. I'd just come downstairs and collapse on the floor. That was in 1987. I was 33 years old. It was just unbelievable pain. I'd go to bed and cry half the night. I didn't feel like a whole person. I had to walk backwards down the stairs, very slowly."

Fast-forward 10 years, to 1998, when Liz began strength training to deal with her arthritis. "I started with leg lifts using free weights—about 3 pounds on each leg. It was hard because my range of motion was really limited. Also, it's so hard to go through the motions when you feel crappy and don't want to move, but the more you do it, the better you feel."

Indeed! Today, Liz strength-trains twice a week. And she does a lot of aerobic exercise, too—both walking and biking. But that's the least of it. As Liz herself says, "Working out has really changed my life. About a year after I first started using weights, I said to the kids, 'Let's go for a hike.' We went to the Camden Hills [a hiking spot in Maine]. Alex, my youngest, said, 'I have never seen you walk like this.' It was amazing to hear that."

Since then, Liz has even climbed Mt. Washington, which, at more than 6,000 feet, is the highest mountain in New England. And she takes 12- to 15-mile bike rides. "I never dreamed that I would be on a bike again," she says. "I have a lot of 'crunch' in my knees. I thought it wasn't an option. Now I say, 'Anything's possible.' There's no question that I have my life back," Liz exclaims. "People I haven't seen for a long time are just amazed at the changes.

My friends will look at me and say, 'Wow, you look so good'. They say I look younger. That makes me feel good. But just the fact that I myself know how much more I can do is what's important."

It's the little things, more than the big hikes and climbs, that Liz particularly marvels over. "So much day-to-day stuff that wasn't part of my life anymore, like pulling wet clothes out of the washing machine, absolutely wrestling with them. It sounds silly to talk about, but it was just so hard to do. And in winter, I'd think, 'Do I really have to go outside today? It's icy. How am I going to negotiate my way to the car?' But now, hauling a 25-pound bag of dog food out of the car and into the house isn't a problem—it's great. I do wish that somebody had said to me along the way, 'The more you move, the better you're going to feel.'"

Think of Liz, who has been there herself, as the person saying that to *you*. But you're already a step ahead. That's because this chapter is an exercise program tailored specifically to *your* needs, whether you have osteoarthritis or rheumatoid arthritis. It's based on the latest scientific evidence about how to help people with either condition regain control of their bodies.

The exercises are all part of a 16-week program. The core exercises—those that you will learn in the first 4 weeks—take less than 30 minutes a day. Additional exercises for increased benefit are added on during the remaining 12 weeks of the program.

All of the exercises illustrated here will both decrease pain and improve your ability to perform everyday tasks and participate in leisure activities. An additional benefit is that the movements will make your body leaner-looking by increasing your muscle mass. That, in turn, makes weight control easier, because muscle burns more calories than fat. The weight-control bonus is particularly important for people with osteoarthritis, since excess weight is a major risk factor for the development and progression of that disease.

ELEMENTS OF THE BEAT ARTHRITIS EXERCISE PROGRAM

There are three types of exercise in our arthritis-fighting program: strength training, flexibility-enhancing moves, and aerobic activities. A combination of all three is crucial for getting optimal results. The strength-training exercises will improve muscle strength (which will relieve stress on the joints), balance, and kinesthetic awareness. That's awareness of one body part in relation to another, for example, how the knee corresponds to the ankle and foot. The aerobic activities will improve cardiovascular fitness—a good thing since the fitness of the heart, lungs, and all the vessels that tie them together is compromised in people with arthritis. The flexibility exercises will allow you to move your limbs through a greater range of motion—to pack away groceries on a high shelf or reach behind you for something. They will also help prevent injuries as you move about.

Strength training

As we explained in Chapter 3, when we conducted a scientific investigation into exercise and knee arthritis at Tufts, we found that strength training just three times a week dramatically improves physical function and decreases pain. It also enables people to become more self-sufficient, improves emotional well-being, and contributes to a better overall outlook on life. It's not surprising when you consider that after just 16 weeks of strength training, the people in our study were significantly stronger, which allowed them to walk, climb stairs, and perform other everyday activities with much more ease. And pain in the knees decreased 43 percent, on average.

Other studies have also confirmed that exercise can lessen pain and improve physical function in people with osteoarthritis of the knee, but the results of many of those studies were—as was the intensity of the training—much more moderate. That's where our program is different: It is designed to help people progress to a high level of intensity—but gradually. The exercises will not only improve your strength but also challenge your balance (and thereby improve it) and require you to think about joint alignment.

The core of the strength-training component of the program is for those with knee arthritis, by far the most common of all types of arthritis. But suggestions for modifications will also be included for those with osteoarthritis of the hand or hip. The program is a balanced one, including exercises for the whole body. Therefore, it is also ideal for those with rheumatoid arthritis, in which multiple joints are affected, and therefore multiple muscles need to be strengthened.

Flexibility exercises

It might seem as though you can dispense with the flexibility part of the exercise program without much harm, but that's not true. It's as important as strength training and aerobic activities. One reason is that optimum flexibility will increase your efficiency of movement. But there's more. Flexibility exercises, which are essentially stretches, decrease stress and tension in the muscles, improve posture, provide relief from muscle cramps and soreness, and decrease the risk for low-back injury and pain.

Flexibility training also relieves *contractures.* Contractures, common in arthritis, are joints that remain partially contracted, even when they're not in use. This shortens a muscle, making it less supple, less strong, and unable to absorb the shock and stress of movements—not what you want when your joints are already under siege. Contractures also cut off circulation to a muscle, inhibiting its supply of oxygen and essential nutrients and allowing waste products to build up in muscle cells.

It's commonly believed that people who engage in strength training develop extra-large muscles and thereby *decrease* their flexibility. But most people,

Dr. Roubenoff sounds off on the benefits of stretching

I can really speak to the importance of stretching from personal experience," Ronenn says. "As a busy physician, I always used to try to squeeze my exercise sessions into as short a time as possible. As a result, I tended to blow off stretching so I could do the *real* exercises—strength training and running. Boy, was that a mistake. It seemed that every few weeks I had a new injury. Finally, I hurt my back badly enough (on the beach, not while training) that I had to lay off my exercise program for 3 months. Then I 'got religion' and started stretching every day. Since then, my injuries have disappeared, and I get much more time for my strength and aerobic training because I'm not spending tons of time nursing injuries!"

save the Arnold Schwarzeneggers of the world, gain a good deal of muscle strength without bulking up. In fact, the size of the muscle does not determine flexibility. If strength-training exercises are done properly, they can actually *enhance* flexibility.

There are two components of proper, flexibility-enhancing strength training: The entire muscle must be worked through its full range of motion, and there must be an emphasis, or mindfulness, on the "negative" phase of each lift. That's the phase during which the weight is being lowered rather than raised, and it's during that phase that the muscle is being stretched and actually has to work harder than it does while lifting the weight.

Aerobic activities

Our program encourages a gradual increase in the duration and intensity of aerobic exercise. We encourage you to include weight-bearing activities as part of your aerobic training. "Weight bearing" means that you carry the weight of your body as you engage in the activity, as in walking. Weight-bearing exercises are required to maintain the integrity of the cartilage in the joint, as is strength training. If your joints are too painful to participate in weight-bearing exercise, choose a non-weight-bearing activity such as swimming or cycling and add weight-bearing exercise as you are able. The aerobic effort will also improve the capacity of your heart and lungs—your cardiovascular system. Improved cardiorespiratory fitness will decrease fatigue in daily activities and decrease the risk for premature death from other chronic diseases, such as heart disease.

A SIXTEEN-WEEK PROGRESSIVE PROGRAM

What we mean by "progressive" is that you start out with just four strength-training exercises and short periods of aerobic activity, both at a low intensity. Some stretching for enhanced flexibility is included from the outset as well. But over the weeks, you will gradually increase the intensity of the workouts as well as incorporate additional exercises. Of course, if you are already physically active you can incorporate the exercises into your current routine.

For the first few weeks, you will spend 30 minutes three times per week doing a combination of strength training, aerobic exercises, and flexibility stretches. By the end of the 16 weeks, the entire strength-training, aerobic, and flexibility program will take you 1 hour and 15 minutes per session if done all at one time. But you don't have to do everything all in the same day. At the end of the chapter we will provide suggestions for exercise routines that can be done in shorter periods of time over 6 days versus longer periods over 3 days. It's simply a matter of splitting up the aerobic and strength training, so you can tailor the program in a way that works for you—or vary it as you go along. However you do it, you need to devote only about 4 hours a week to exercise once you get up to speed—not much when you consider that a week has 168 hours in it.

As with anything, the more you put into the program, the more you will get out of it. But the most important thing with exercise is consistency. You have to keep doing it over the long run. Individualize the program according to what is realistic for you in terms of time commitment and motivation. Always start with what you know you can handle, and build on it as you go.

Before you get started

Unfortunately, a lot of people don't go for a once-a-year checkup at the doctor's. It's understandable. Why go looking for bad news, especially if you're feeling okay?

Anything you find out in an annual physical is *good* news. Even if you turn out to have a serious medical problem, the earlier it's caught, the better the chance your doctor has of treating it effectively. And if you find out that you've got a clean bill of health, which most people do, you can breathe easy and not have to wonder whether there may be something wrong that your body isn't telling you with obvious symptoms.

For those reasons, if you haven't been examined by a doctor in at least a year, we strongly advise you to just pick up the phone and schedule a physical. As an added precaution, take the PAR-Q (Physical Activity Readiness Questionnaire) on the pages that follow to determine whether you should be aware of any cautions as you start the exercise program. Nearly everyone can conduct the exercises safely, but by taking the PAR-Q, you're playing it extra safe.

If you're in any doubt about your physical readiness, check with your doctor during your physical—your doctor knows you best, and he or she can advise you as to whether it is safe to start an exercise program. If you're over age 70, check with your doctor regardless of your PAR-Q score.

Gear

Most of the equipment you will need can be found at a sporting goods store, although there are also a number of mail-order sources. See "Resources" at the back of the book for those.

Dumbbells

To start the program you will need pairs of 1-, 2-, 3- and 5-pound dumbbells. (No need to buy 1- and 2-pound dumbbells. You can use the 1-pound pellets from the ankle weights.) As you get stronger you will need pairs of 8-, 10-, 12-, and maybe 15-pound dumbbells. Buy them as you become stronger and need them. Expect to pay about sixty cents per pound for each dumbbell. This means that a 5-pound dumbbell costs about three dollars. There are some dumbbells available that are adjustable—just make sure that you try them out and that they are comfortable to hold and easy to adjust. If you have difficulty gripping the dumbbells because of your arthritis, buy adjustable wrist weights that fit snuggly around your wrists.

Ankle weights

Starting at week 9, you will be using ankle weights—strap-on cuffs with "pockets" that hold weighted bars. You adjust the weight of the cuff by adding or removing bars. There are two sizes of weights you can buy: ones with cuffs that hold 20 pounds and ones with cuffs that hold 10 pounds. We recommend buying the 20-pound cuffs because, for one of the exercises, most people can progress to more than 10 pounds per leg. That's a lot of weight, but keep in mind that you can start with as little as 1 pound and keep adding weight as you become stronger. Ten-pound ankle weights cost about thirty dollars each; 20-pound cuffs cost about fifty dollars each. You can buy just one cuff. However, the routine will take longer because you'll have to switch it from leg to leg.

Physical Activity Readiness
Questionnare—PAR-Q
(revised 1994)

PAR-Q & YOU
(A Questionnaire for People Aged 15 to 69)

Regular physical activity is fun and healthy, and increasingly more people are starting to become more active every day. Being more active is very safe for most people. However, some people should check with their doctor before they start becoming much more physically active.

If you are planning to become much more physically active than you are now, start by answering the seven questions in the box below. If you are between the ages of 15 and 69, the PAR-Q will tell you if you should check with your doctor before you start. If you are over 69 years of age, and you are not used to being very active, check with your doctor.

Common sense is your best guide when you answer these questions. Please read the questions carefully and answer each one honestly: check YES or NO.

YES	NO		
☐	☐	1.	Has your doctor ever said that you have a heart condition <u>and</u> that you should only do physical activity recommended by a doctor?
☐	☐	2.	Do you feel pain in your chest when you do physical activity?
☐	☐	3.	In the past month, have you had chest pain when you were not doing physical activity?
☐	☐	4.	Do you lose your balance because of dizziness or do you ever lose consciousness?
☐	☐	5.	Do you have a bone or joint problem that could be made worse by a change in your physical activity?
☐	☐	6.	Is your doctor currently prescribing drugs (for example, water pills) for your blood pressure or heart condition?
☐	☐	7.	Do you know of <u>any other reason</u> why you should not do physical activity?

**IF
YOU
ANSWERED**

YES to one or more questions

Talk with your doctor by phone or in person BEFORE you start becoming much more physically active or BEFORE you have a fitness appraisal. Tell your doctor about the PAR-Q and which questions you answered YES.

- You may be able to do any activity you want—as long as you start slowly and build up gradually. Or, you may need to restrict your activities to those which are safe for you. Talk with your doctor about the kinds of activities you wish to participate in and follow his/her advice.
- Find out which community programs are safe and helpful for you.

NO to all questions

If you answered NO honestly to <u>all</u> PAR-Q questions, you can be reasonably sure that you can:

- start becoming much more physically active—begin slowly and build up gradually. This is the safest and easiest way to go.
- take part in a fitness appraisal—this is an excellent way to determine your basic fitness so that you can plan the best way for you to live actively.

DELAY BECOMING MUCH MORE ACTIVE:

- if you are not feeling well because of a temporary illness such as a cold or fever—wait until you feel better; or
- if you are or may be pregnant—talk to your doctor before you start becoming more active.

Please note: If your health changes so that you then answer YES to any of the above questions, tell your fitness or health professional. Ask whether you should change your physical activity plan.

<u>Informed Use of the PAR-Q:</u> The Canadian Society for Exercise Physiology, Health Canada, and their agents assume no liability for persons who undertake physical activity, and if in doubt after completing this questionnaire, consult your doctor prior to physical activity.

Chair

Select a sturdy chair. The seat of the chair should be long enough to support your legs from the buttocks to the backs of the knees. The chair should also be high enough so that the soles of your shoes just barely touch the floor. You can adjust the height with seat cushions.

Staircase or step

One of the exercises requires a staircase or an exercise step. If you don't have access to a staircase with a handrail, you can purchase a step. Exercise steps are available at sporting goods stores, but they can be relatively expensive—about fifty dollars. A less expensive alternative—ten to twenty dollars—is a sturdy utility stool 8–12 inches high, which you can find at a hardware store or good department store. Make sure that the step has four solid legs and a skid-proof top and that it can hold your body weight easily without tipping over.

Exercise mat (optional)

A firm exercise mat makes floor exercises more comfortable. You can also use a large bath towel. Place the towel or mat on a rug, if possible, for added cushioning.

What to wear

Wear loose, nonrestrictive clothing that will not cause you to overheat. Also wear sturdy supportive shoes that are not worn out, preferably athletic shoes. Here is a check to determine if your shoes are too worn. Place your shoes on a table or counter at eye level and determine if the soles are worn on the outside or inside edges. You may see wear in the soles on either side and/or in the heel of the shoe, leaning in or out. Exercising with shoes that are worn out can overstress the joints. That's true of all the shoes you wear, not just the ones in which you work out. Another rule of thumb: If you have been using one pair of athletic shoes for a year, it is time to replace them.

Water

Water should be an integral part of your workout gear. Have a bottle of water handy, and drink half a cup every 15–20 minutes. Also drink a cup an hour before and shortly after you work out. Plenty of fluid will allow your body to perform and adapt optimally.

Stand tall with good posture

Good posture is key to minimizing the stress on your joints—as well as stress on the spine. Good posture will also reduce muscle strain and injury. Read over the following guidelines for good posture and follow them not only in your exercise regimen but also in your daily activities.

Posture begins with the feet. How the feet are positioned affects the alignment of the ankles, knees, hips, and spine. When the feet are unbalanced, the body is unsupported and subject to stress. Good positioning of your feet will translate up your body.

When standing for any length of time, keep weight evenly distributed on both feet. Many people with arthritis in one knee or hip will compensate by putting more weight on the other side. This is a natural response, and it is often effective at relieving pain—at first. But over time, the pressure on the "good" leg grows to the point that it, too, develops arthritis. The better solution is to strengthen the muscles in both legs, but especially the more severely affected one. That's the way to protect the joints in the long run.

Note that many people with osteoarthritis of the knee turn their feet outward when they walk in order to relieve pain. However, this causes the inner arches of the foot to collapse. It also pulls the pelvis forward and stresses the spine, often causing backache.

How to Stand with Good Posture

- Keep feet hip-width (12 inches) apart.
- The outside of your feet should form two parallel lines. It may make you feel pigeon toed until you get used to it.
- Keep your toes on the ground. Stretch them forward as if trying to extend the soles of your feet. It's more a feeling than an actual movement.
- Keep your weight evenly distributed between your two feet.
- Keep your knees straight but not locked.
- Pull your tailbone under you slightly.
- Keep your shoulders drawn back and down. This will lift and broaden your chest. You should feel comfortable in the shoulders.
- Your chin should be parallel with the ground.
- Think of a string attached to the top of your head lifting you up.

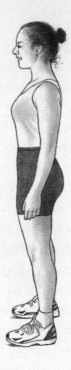

Warm up and cool down

Most injuries to muscle and connective tissue occur when the body has not been adequately prepared for the stress of exercise, so you should always prepare your body for physical activity. That means doing 3–5 minutes of low-intensity walking, dancing, calisthenics, or riding a stationary bike to warm up. You can choose a warm-up activity that mimics one in your workout, but do it at a lower intensity (for instance, walking before you start jogging). This low-intensity activity will prepare your motor-skill coordinating system and heighten your kinesthetic awareness. Another benefit of a warm-up, no matter which one you choose, is increased blood supply, and therefore an increase in nutrients flowing to the muscles. This will increase the lubrication in your joints as well as muscle and tendon elasticity, which in turn decreases the chance of injury.

A proper cool-down is also critical for a safe and effective workout. The cool-down allows your body to recover safely by slowly returning to its resting state. Your heart rate will gradually decrease and your blood pressure will normalize, which is important for cardiovascular health. Five minutes of light activity, just as in warming up, will suffice for a cool-down. Stretching happens to be a great way to cool down after strength training because the activity helps to further improve flexibility, which reduces your risk for injury.

STRENGTH TRAINING: GENERAL GUIDELINES

The key to improving strength is to challenge your muscles to the point that they adapt to the extra load and become stronger. If the challenge, or load, is not great enough, the muscle will not respond and strengthen; if the challenge is *too* great, you risk injuring the muscle and surrounding joints and tissues. The success of our program is that it is tailored to training at the proper intensity so that it provides you with an appropriate challenge for improving strength. And you can keep progressing to maintain that intensity as your muscles adapt and become stronger—which helps to continually lessen symptoms.

When you train at a high enough intensity to strengthen your muscles, microscopic muscle fibers break down—a harmless, and even necessary, part of the strengthening process. But if your body cannot adequately recover from the microtears, the system will falter, and you will not progress. So it is important once you are training at the recommended intensity that you rest the muscles you used in a workout for at least one day before working them again. (That's not the case for flexibility and aerobic exercises, which will be discussed later.) In addition, people with severe rheumatoid cachexia may need *two* days' rest between workouts.

Reps and sets

In strength training, a single, complete move is called a *repetition*, or *rep*. If you can do 15 or more reps easily, you are improving your muscular endurance more than your strength. If you are able to do fewer than 15 and feel that you've reached your limit when you are done, you are improving your muscular strength. *That's the goal.* In our program, 12 reps make a *set*, and you do two sets of each exercise at a time, with a short rest between them.

At the proper intensity, you should find the weight moderately difficult to lift the first time, but well within your capability. By the sixth or seventh repetition, it should seem heavier. Ideally, you should be able to perform the twelfth rep in good form but feel that if you didn't stop and rest your muscles, you couldn't continue.

How to evaluate your effort

The following scale—inspired by the Borg Intensity Scale used by many researchers—will help you evaluate the intensity of each strength-training exercise. For each exercise, evaluate your intensity at the end of 2 sets of 12 repetitions.

Finding the right challenge and progression

At the beginning of the program and whenever a new exercise is introduced, the intensity of the exercise should be a three or less. That will allow you to perfect your form and give your muscles time to become familiar with each exercise. Once your form is perfected, the goal over the next few workouts is

EXERCISE INTENSITY SCALE FOR STRENGTH TRAINING	
EXERCISE INTENSITY	DESCRIPTION OF EFFORT
1	*Very easy:* Too easy to be noticed, like lifting a pencil.
2	*Easy:* Can be felt but isn't fatiguing, like carrying a book.
3	*Moderate:* Fatiguing only if prolonged, like carrying a full handbag that seems heavier as the day goes on.
4	*Hard:* More than moderate at first, and becoming difficult by the time you complete 6 or 7 repetitions. You can make the effort 12 times in good form, but need to rest afterward.
5	*Extremely hard:* Requires all your strength, like lifting a piece of heavy furniture that you can only lift once, if at all.

to increase the intensity to a four. This is the proper intensity for improving strength.

Progressions are provided for each exercise, meaning that you go from lower to greater intensity. Everyone should start with the first progression until the form is mastered. If the first progression starts out feeling like a four on the intensity scale, do fewer than 12 repetitions. When the form is mastered, increase to 12 repetitions.

Increase one progression per workout. If the progression is to increase the weight you are lifting, increase the weight by one increment per workout. As you become stronger, the intensity will drop below a four again. At that point, proceed once again through the next progression. (This will become clearer once you read through the exercises and begin the program.)

You may find that your muscles are sore after the first few workouts at an intensity of four. This is normal. In fact, it is a sign that you are challenging your muscles appropriately to adapt and become stronger. The soreness should not be to the point where daily activities become bothersome or difficult. If that is the case, move down one progression.

Try to increase the progression every couple of weeks in the second and third months or until you have reached the top progression. Don't worry if it's not always possible. You'll soon see that progress is easier with some exercises than with others. Don't be discouraged—all of your muscle groups will become stronger if you persist. The key to strength training is to begin slowly and progress consistently.

How to do the exercises

Don't forget to warm up before you strength-train, just as you would before doing aerobics, by doing 3–5 minutes of light activity. The activity may be the squat or stair-stepping exercise described below, done at a very easy intensity for a couple of minutes, or you may take a brisk walk around the block. You will cool down at the end of the strength program with the flexibility exercises that are described later.

Timing

The timing of each repetition is important. It ensures that the muscle—not gravity or momentum—is doing the work. A single lift should take about 8 seconds: 3 seconds to raise the weight, a 1-second pause, and 4 seconds to return to the starting position. Then there is a pause while you take a breath before starting the next repetition.

Remember, if you are working at an intensity of four, at the end of 12 repetitions you should have to rest. Rest 30 seconds–1 minute between sets. The rest increases blood flow to the muscle, washing away metabolic waste products and preventing injury. Rest is not a waste of time; it's an active part of the training, even if it seems like doing nothing.

For each exercise, a brief description that outlines the muscles to be targeted is provided. It is important to focus on these muscles and actually visualize them contracting to lift and stretching to lower from the lift. While the muscles performing the exercise will be tensing up, it is important not to tense other muscles in the body. In the middle of each lift, during the one-second pause, you should scan your body for tension in areas other than the muscles being worked—and relax them.

Breathe when you do the exercises—*do not hold your breath.* It is crucial that you exhale as you lift the weight and inhale as you lower it, even though that is the opposite of what most people would do intuitively. Failing to breathe can raise your blood pressure too much as you lift the weight, reducing the blood flow to your muscles. It can also increase your risk for hernias and other injuries. If you can't get the correct rhythm when you first start, don't worry. Just make sure that you are breathing throughout the move. As you become more comfortable with the exercises, you will be able to incorporate the correct breathing rhythm.

Alternatively, until the exercises become comfortable, count aloud the 8 seconds of each rep. This will make you breathe and do the exercise at the appropriate speed.

Caution: Always take precautions when you are moving your weights or any heavy objects. Use your legs, not your back, to lift heavy things, keeping the knees flexed, back straight, and body close to the object. Don't swoop down in a back-bending motion to lift something; bend your legs so your back stays in position.

Stage 1: Weeks 1–4

Begin with these four strengthening exercises. You will not need weights at the beginning. (Note: If you have osteoarthritis of the hip, check out the modifications beginning on page 122.)

MODIFIED SQUAT ◆

This is a multijoint exercise that will strengthen the inner, front, and back of the thighs and the buttock muscles, mitigating arthritis pain. Strengthening these muscles will make it easier to walk, climb stairs and hills, get up from a chair, and in and out of a car. The exercise requires balance and awareness of the alignment of back, hips, knees, and ankles, working your lower-body muscles in a way that is consistent with how they are used in daily activities.

Starting position: Stand in front of a chair with your back to it and your feet slightly further apart than hip-width and toes pointed out slightly. Cross your arms over your chest and pull your shoulders back and down (in a relaxed position). Focus your eyes on an object in front of you at eye level. Lean forward slightly from the hips, keeping your back straight. Pull in your abdominal muscles slightly to support your back. Avoid overarching your lower back. Evenly distribute your body weight from the balls of your feet to the heels, and also on your feet's outer and inner edges.

E
X
E
R
C
I
S
E
S

1-2-3-Down: Bending at the hip, slowly lower your buttocks back toward the chair seat, maintaining your upper-body posture.

Pause for a second.

1-2-Up: Push up from the chair with the same posture and positioning. Do not lock your knees at the top of the movement.

Reps and sets: Repeat the move until you have done 12 repetitions—this is 1 set. Rest for about 30 seconds and then do a second set.

Focal points: Do not bend further at the waist as you descend, and keep your chest lifted and pointing forward. As you lower yourself into the chair, do not let your knees come in front of your toes—you will need to push out your buttocks. Keep each knee in line with the middle toe. Do not let the knees go in toward each other (knock kneed) or drift away (bow legged). Proper alignment makes all the difference in avoiding stress on the knees when squatting or, as in the next exercise, climbing stairs.

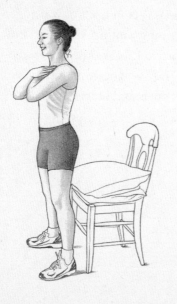
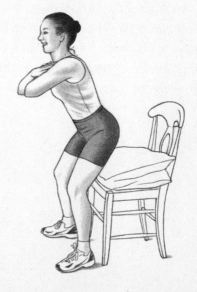

Progressions

1. If you cannot get out of the chair as described above in a slow, smooth, controlled form, start by placing a firm pillow or two or folded blanket on the chair to raise you up. Raise the level of the chair until you can perform the move in a slow, smooth, controlled manner.

2. Complete the exercise without the cushions or blankets for 2 sets of 12. If 2 sets is too difficult for this progression, do the first set with cushions and try the second set without. Work up to 2 sets without the cushions or blankets.

3. On the descent, do not sit in the chair but instead just tap the chair with your buttocks without taking your weight off your legs and feet, and then push back up to the starting position. Again, if 2 sets are too difficult, you may progress by doing the first set tapping the chair and the second set pausing in the seated position before rising.

4. Hold a 5-pound dumbbell in each hand while performing the exercise as described above. Keep hands down at your sides. Continue to maintain your upper-body posture for the exercise when using dumbbells. Progress to 8 pounds, 10 pounds, and 12 pounds as you get stronger.

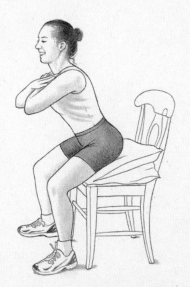

STEP-UP ◆

This is also a multijoint exercise that will strengthen the muscles on the fronts and backs of your thighs as well as on your hips. Like the squat, it will improve balance, coordination, and spatial awareness. It will make it easier to walk and climb stairs and hills.

Starting position: Stand 1–1½ feet in front of a staircase or step, with feet hip-width apart. Stand tall with your back straight, shoulders back and down, and head in line with your spine. Focus your eyes on an object straight ahead at eye level. Place your left foot completely on the step with a slight forward lean in your trunk. Lean from the hips; do not bend at the waist. Your left knee should be over your ankle and perpendicular to the floor.

1-2-Up: Pull up and forward with your left leg to bring your right foot up to the step.

Tap the toes of the right foot on the stair and pause for 1 second.

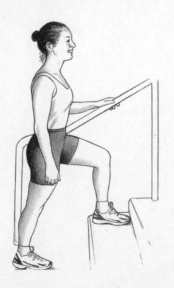 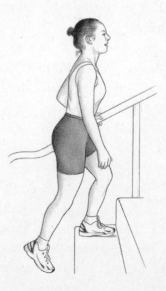

1-2-3-Down: Step back off with the right foot. Your left leg will be controlling the descent. The left foot remains on the step until you have completed all the repetitions for that leg. Then switch and place your right foot on the stair and repeat.

Reps and sets: Repeat the move 12 times on each side—this is 1 set. Rest for about 30 seconds and then do a second set.

Focal points: Do not let your leading knee go in front of your toes. Keep your trunk erect and your neck in line with your trunk during the movement. Do not bend at the waist on the way up or down. The more you pull up with the leg on the step, the more you will feel both the front and back of the leg working—which is just what you want.

Progressions
1. Start with a 7- to 8-inch step with a railing. If you cannot step up in a smooth, controlled motion with good form, use the handrail to assist in ascending and descending. You should use the handrail only for balance—don't grip it tightly. When you use the handrail, do not change the form of the exercise.
2. Use a 7- to 8-inch step with no assist from the hands.
3. Go to two steps on your staircase or a 15-i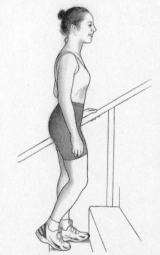 step. At this height your knee will form a 90-d angle, and your thigh will be parallel to the flc Do not use a step that places your knee at less than a 90-degree angle.
4. Do the exercise as described above, but hold a 5-pound dumbbell in each hand, keeping your hands down at your side at hip level. Continue to maintain proper form in the upper body when using dumbbells. Only progress to this level if you feel safe and comfortable.

TOE STAND ◆

This exercise will strengthen your calf muscles and improve the mobility of your ankles. Loss of ankle mobility is common with arthritis and can affect your ability to walk and climb stairs.

Starting position: Stand approximately 1 foot behind the back of the chair with your feet hip-width apart, knees slightly bent. Keep your back straight, your head in line with your spine, and your shoulders back and down. Use the chair for balance—don't lean on the chair.

1-2-Up: Raise your heels off the floor, pushing straight up onto the balls of your feet. Go as high as you can.

Pause for a second or two.

1-2-3-Down: Slowly lower your heels to the starting position.

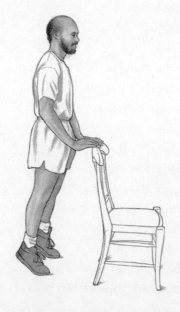

Reps and sets: Repeat the move until you have done 12 repetitions—this is 1 set. Rest for about 30 seconds and then do a second set.

Focal points: Spread the weight evenly across your toes. Do not let your ankles fall in or out. Keep your trunk erect and knees slightly bent during the movement.

Progressions

1. The first goal is to work on the height to which you can raise your heels off the floor. Work to raise your heels at least 3 inches off the floor.

2. Place the balls of your feet on the bottom step of a stair. For balance, hold on to the rail of the stairs. With the same posture as above, complete the heel lift, but on the descent, let your heels drop below the step. The ascent from this position will be more challenging, and you will be working the ankle through a greater range of motion.

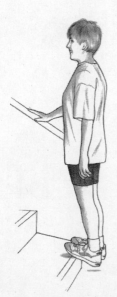 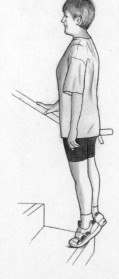

Progression 2

MODIFIED PUSH-UP ◆

Push-ups are great because they do not require any equipment (you use your body weight for resistance), and they work multiple muscle groups, including those in the chest, shoulders, backs of your upper arms, and trunk. Increasing the strength in your chest will improve your strength for any movements you do with your arms. The chest is the core of your upper-body strength. By varying the form, you will use more or less of your body weight to control the intensity.

Starting position: Stand about 3 feet back from a wall. Lean forward toward the wall, keeping your ankles, knees, hips, shoulders, and head in a straight line. Position your hands at shoulder height on the wall with your fingers spread and pointing toward the ceiling. Arms should be straight without locking the elbows.

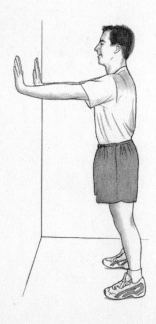 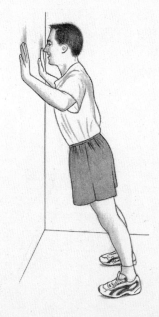

1-2-3-Down: Bend your elbows and lower your body toward the wall, keeping your body in a straight line.

When your nose is near the wall, pause for 1 second.

1-2-Up: Push back to the starting position.

Reps and sets: Repeat the move until you have done 12 repetitions—this is 1 set. Rest for about 30 seconds and then do a second set.

Focal points: Do not bend at the waist to reach the wall. Pull in your abdominal muscles slightly to avoid arching your lower back. As you push back from the wall, visualize your chest muscles squeezing together. If you have trouble with your wrists when pushing from the wall try wearing oven mitts or putting a folded towel between you and the wall to act as a cushion. Or you can try making fists and pushing off with your knuckles.

Progressions
1. Wall push-up as described above.
2. Same push-up as above, but place your hands on the edge of a counter or sturdy desk instead of on a wall. You will lift more of your body weight in this position. Maintain a straight body as you lower and raise, as you did using the wall. Do not bend at the waist to reach the desk; that lessens the amount of body weight you are supporting.

Stage 2: Weeks 5–8

Add the following two exercises. These are trunk exercises that are important for your posture. They also provide a strong base of support for your limbs. Strengthening your limbs without strengthening your trunk muscles not only will set you up for a back injury but also will limit the improvements you can make. The trunk muscles support all movements.

For these exercises you will not perform 2 sets of 12 repetitions, as you do for the other strength exercises. You will obtain the best results if you concentrate on precise form and hold the pose or position for a longer and longer time as described under "Progressions." You will do 5 repetitions and build up the time you hold the position.

BACK EXTENSION ◆

This exercise is a yoga pose that will strengthen the back and buttock muscles, which will greatly improve your posture and relieve any stress you may have in your lower back. The stronger your trunk muscles, the more you can use them to help arthritic joints in the limbs.

Starting position: Lie face down with your forehead resting on the floor, legs stretched back, toes pointing back. Stretch back your arms on either side of your body, palms facing up. Tuck your tailbone under you slightly (same motion as pushing your pubic bone into the floor).

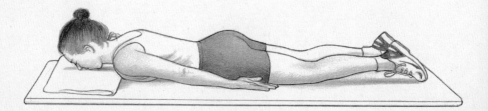

1-2-Up: As you inhale, raise your chest off the floor, keeping your head, neck, and back all in line.

Hold the position for 3–5 seconds.

1-2-3-Down: Exhale as you lower back to the ground.

Sets and reps: Repeat the movement until you have done 5 repetitions. Rest for 15 seconds between each repetition.

Focal points: Think of extending up rather than crunching through the lower back. Keep your shoulders back and your chest broadening as you rise up and lower down.

Progressions
1. Hold the lifted position for 3–5 seconds.
2. Hold for 10 seconds.
3. Increase hold for 20 seconds.

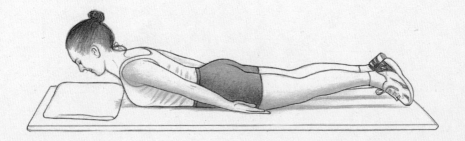

MODIFIED BOAT POSE ◆

This exercise will strengthen the abdominal muscles. The abdominal muscles, along with the back extension muscles trained in the previous exercise, form the scaffolding that holds up your trunk. In addition, strengthening the abdominal muscles firms the tummy.

Starting position and movement: Sit on the floor with your legs straight out in front of you and your hands behind your back, fingers pointing forward, to help support your back. Bend your knees, keeping your feet on the floor. Lift and open your chest by pulling your shoulders back and down, and pull your tailbone underneath you. Take as much weight off your hands as possible without slouching/rounding your back, balancing on the front of your buttocks. Hold the position for 3–5 seconds.

Sets and reps: Repeat the move until you have done 5 repetitions. Rest for 15 seconds between repetitions.

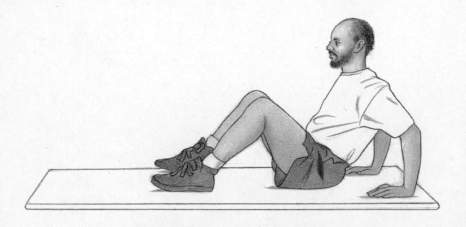

Focal points: Think of extending up through your trunk. Keep your shoulders back and your chest broadening as you hold the pose.

Progressions

1. Hold the lifted position for 3–5 seconds, using your hands on the floor to support your trunk if necessary.

2. Hold for 10–20 seconds without the use of your hands, as illustrated below.

3. Raise your feet and hands off the floor while you balance on your buttocks. Start with 5 repetitions of 10 seconds each and then progress to 5 repetitions of 20 seconds each.

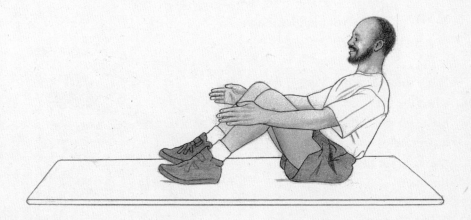

Stage 3: Weeks 9–12

Add the following two exercises to your routine. They really target the muscles of your thighs and therefore are important for relieving arthritis pain, especially for those with knee or hip osteoarthritis, where the thigh muscles are weak. You will need your ankle weights for them.

KNEE EXTENSION ◆

This exercise works the front thigh muscles, or quadriceps. The quadriceps have been shown to be the weakest link in individuals with osteoarthritis of the knee, so it's important to include an exercise that isolates and targets these weak muscles by themselves. You will need a chair, possibly a cushion, and your ankle weights.

Starting position: Sit with your back and hips against the back of the chair. If necessary, utilize pillows, folded blankets, or cushions to increase the height of the chair so that only your toes are resting on the ground. Start with your knees bent at 90 degrees.

1-2-Up: Extend your left leg out as straight as possible.

Pause for 1 second when the leg is as high as you can lift it pain free, or when the leg is parallel to the floor.

1-2-3-Down: Lower your left leg back to the starting position.

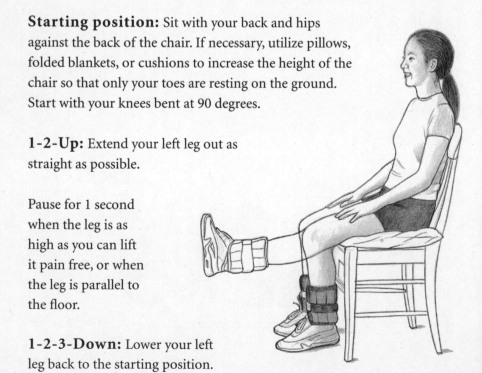

Reps and sets: Complete 12 repetitions on one side and then repeat on the other side—this is 1 set. Rest for about 30 seconds and then do a second set.

Focal points: Keep your back against the back of the chair and your hips down during the movement; you don't want to arch your back as you do the move. Keep your toes pointing toward the ceiling and in line with the knee during the movement. Visualize the thigh muscles doing the work and relax your other muscles, especially those in the calves.

Progressions

1. Women should start with 3 pounds in each ankle weight, men 3–5 pounds. Increase the weight by 1–2 pounds with each workout until you are at four on the intensity scale. If the weight seems too difficult at first, do the move without the ankle weights until the move is comfortable.

2. Continue increasing the weight by 1–2 pounds as you become stronger in order to maintain the intensity at a four.

3. To increase the difficulty of the move and better isolate the different muscles of the upper thigh, try varying the foot position. Point foot "in" for 4 repetitions, foot "straight" for 4 repetitions, and then foot "out" for the final 4 repetitions of each set. The rotation of the foot comes from the hip, not the ankle.

KNEE FLEXION ◆

This exercise will strengthen the muscles in the back of the thigh, called the *hamstrings*. Because it is important to balance the strength between the quadriceps and the hamstrings to avoid knee injury and to reduce knee pain, this move is always done in conjunction with the knee extension.

Starting position: Stand up straight with your head in line with your spine, legs hip-width apart, and knees slightly bent as you face a chair (or stand next to a counter). Rest your hands on the chair and use only for balance, not to support your weight. Do not lean or bend forward from the waist or hips.

1-2-Up: Maintaining good posture, raise your left heel toward your buttocks as high as you can or until your calf is parallel to the floor. Make sure throughout the move that you keep both thighs parallel to each other—don't move one in front of the other.

Pause for 1 second.

1-2-3-Down: Lower the left leg to the ground.

Reps and sets: Complete 12 repetitions on one side and then repeat on the other side—this is 1 set. Rest for about 30 seconds and then do a second set.

Focal points: Keep the knee of the supporting leg slightly bent. Keep your

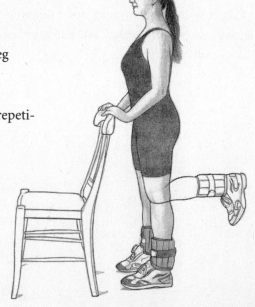

torso erect, and do not arch your back during the lift. Do not let the knee of the working leg come forward of the hip. Try to relax your calf as you raise your leg. The toes of the working leg should be pointing toward the ground.

Progressions

1. Women should start with 1 pound in each ankle weight, men with 3 pounds. Increase the weight by 1–2 pounds with each workout until you are at four on the intensity scale. If the weight seems too difficult at first, do the move without the ankle weights until the move is comfortable.

2. Continue increasing the weight by 1–2 pounds per workout as you become stronger in order to maintain the intensity at a four.

Stage 4: Weeks 13–16

Add the following exercises for more upper-body strength. You will need 1-, 2-, 3-, and 5-pound dumbbells for these moves. If you were using the ankle weights before, you can use the 1-pound pellets to begin with and then tape two 1-pound pellets together for 2-pound weights. This helps to reduce the cost of the lower weights, since you only have to buy 3- and 5-pound dumbbells to start.

REVERSE FLY ◆

This exercise will strengthen the muscles of the upper back and shoulders. Strength in these muscles will prevent slouching in the upper body, thereby eliminating stress on the spine. Strong upper back and shoulders will also help support arthritic joints in the arms and back.

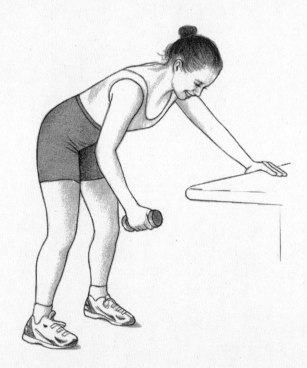

Starting position: Stand several feet back from a table, feet shoulder-width apart. Bend forward from the hips toward the table so that your back is just shy of being parallel to the floor. Rest your left hand on the table, and let your right arm hang straight down with palm facing in.

1-2-Up: Raise your right arm directly out to the side, keeping your elbow relaxed and palm facing down. Think of your shoulder as a hinge throughout the move.

Pause for 1 second when you cannot raise any higher without hunching your shoulder or the right arm is at shoulder height.

1-2-3-Down: Lower your arm to the starting position.

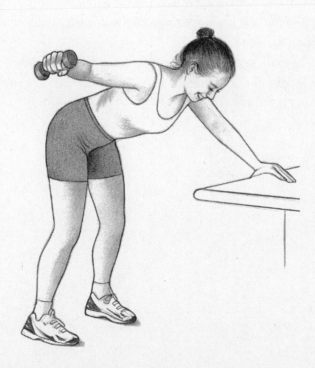

Reps and sets: Complete 12 repetitions with one arm and then switch and complete 12 repetitions with the other one—this is 1 set. Rest for about 30 seconds and then do a second set.

Focal points: Do not lean forward toward the table. Instead, bend from the hips, keeping your legs straight. Think of a pole running up your ankle, knee, and hip, perpendicular to the floor. You, not the table, should be supporting most of your body weight. Keep your back straight and your neck in line with your spine. Initiate the move in the back of your shoulder, and visualize the right shoulder blade squeezing toward the left shoulder blade. Do not hunch your shoulder as you lift, and keep your elbow in line with your shoulder and wrist. When holding the weight, keep your wrist neutral—avoid letting the weight bring the wrist into extension or flexion.

Progressions

1. Practice the exercise without weight until you can do 12 repetitions in good form. At this point start with a 1-pound weight and increase the weight by 1–3 pounds per workout until the intensity is a four after 2 sets of 12 repetitions.

2. As you become stronger and the intensity decreases below a four, increase the weight of the dumbbells by 1–3 pounds each workout until you reach a four on the intensity scale.

LATERAL SHOULDER RAISE ◆

This exercise strengthens the front and middle portions of the shoulder and the upper back. Along with the reverse fly, it helps to tone and strengthen your entire shoulder joint and back, ensuring good posture and upper-body strength.

Starting position: Sit on the front edge of a chair with feet shoulder-width apart. With dumbbells in each hand, hang your arms down at your sides, palms facing toward the chair and with a slight bend in your elbows. Sit tall, with your back straight and your head in line with your spine.

1-2-Up: Raise up both arms to shoulder height, keeping your elbows soft and palms facing down. Maintain the slight bend in your elbows throughout the move.

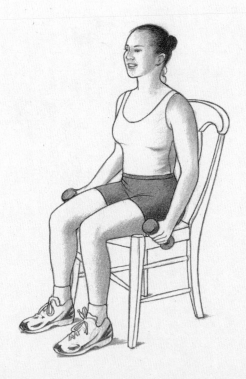

Pause for 1 second.

1-2-3-Down: Return to the starting position.

Reps and sets: Repeat the move until you have done 12 repetitions—this is 1 set. Rest for about 30 seconds and then do a second set.

Focal points: Keep your upper body stable, and do not arch your lower back as you lift. Initiate the movement in the shoulders, but do not hunch up your shoulders as you lift. Keep your shoulders relaxed. When holding the dumbbells, keep your wrist neutral. Avoid letting the weight bring the wrist into extension or flexion.

Variation: Try this variation if you have any shoulder or elbow pain while doing this exercise. Change the rotation of the arms in the starting position

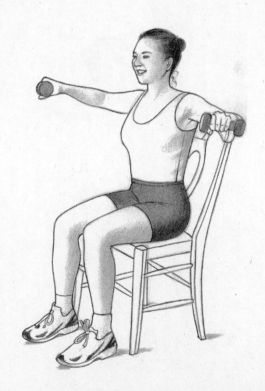

so that the palms face forward. Maintain the rotation throughout the lift; do not change it as you lift. Experiment with how much rotation is needed to perform the exercise pain free.

Progressions

1. Practice the exercise without weight until you can do 12 repetitions in good form. Then start with a 1- to 3-pound weight in each hand and increase the weight by 1–3 pounds per workout until the intensity is a four on the scale after 2 sets of 12 repetitions.

2. As you become stronger and the intensity decreases below a four, increase the weight of the dumbbells by 1- to 3-pound increments per workout to reach a four on the intensity scale.

OSTEOARTHRITIS OF THE HIP

If you have hip arthritis and you find that weight-bearing exercises such as the squat and step-up are too painful, modify the program as follows.

Stage 1: Weeks 1–4

HIP EXTENSION ◆

This exercise will strengthen the hamstrings and buttocks (gluteal muscles), muscles that surround the hip joint. Strength in these muscles is required for getting out of a chair and climbing stairs and hills.

Starting position: Lie on the floor on your stomach with legs extended, toes pointing down. Place your arms in front of your head, and rest your head on your hands with your forehead facing down. *Note:* You can use a firm bed for this exercise if you are unable to get down on the floor.

1-2-Up: Raise your right leg from your hip joint, keeping your leg straight and your trunk stable, toes pointing down toward the ground.

Pause for 1 second when you feel a squeeze in the buttock muscle. (If you feel any pain or a pinch in your lower back, you have lifted the leg too high. Lower it slightly until the feeling in your back subsides.)

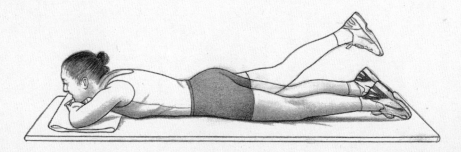

1-2-3-Down: Lower your right leg to the floor.

Reps and sets: Complete 12 repetitions on one side and then repeat on the other side—this is 1 set. Rest for about 30 seconds and then do a second set.

Focal points: Keep your upper body still and relaxed during the exercise. Relax your calf muscle. Initiate the movement from your hip and the back of your thigh. Visualize the hamstrings and buttocks contracting to lift the leg.

Progressions
1. Practice the exercise without ankle weights until you can do 12 repetitions in good form. Then increase the weight by 1-pound increments per workout with ankle weights until you are at a four on the scale.
2. As you become stronger and the intensity falls below a four, increase the weight by 1- to 2-pound increments each workout until you are at a four again.

HIP ABDUCTION ◆

This exercise will strengthen the muscles on the outer thighs and
hips. These muscles are important for balance, walking, running, and
climbing. Strong outer and inner thigh muscles help stabilize the hip,
decreasing stress on the joint.

Starting position: Lie on the floor on your right side with your left leg
extended and your right leg bent at a 90-degree angle at the knee, with your
foot behind you. Align your shoulders, knees, and hips perpendicular to the
floor. Support your head with your right hand. Place your left hand on the
floor in front of you for balance. *Note:* You can use a firm bed for this exercise if you are unable to get down on the floor.

1-2-Up: Raise your left leg from the hip, keeping your trunk stable and
toes pointing forward. Work toward raising your leg to where it forms a
45-degree angle with the floor. At first you may only be able to lift it about
12 inches.

Pause for 1 second.

1-2-3-Down: Lower your leg to the starting position.

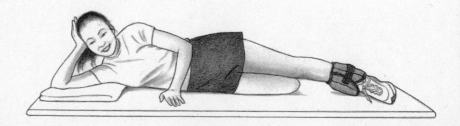

Reps and sets: Do 12 repetitions on one side, rest, and repeat. Then position yourself on your left side and do 2 sets of 12 repetitions for the right leg.

Focal points: Do not lean forward or backward during the movement. Keep your body in a straight line. Relax your upper body and your lower leg during the lift. Initiate the movement from the hip, and visualize the outer hip muscle contracting as you lift.

Progressions

1. Start without any weight. When you can do 12 repetitions in good form, increase the weight by 1-pound increments until you are at a four on the intensity scale for 2 sets of 12 repetitions.

2. As you become stronger and the intensity falls below a four, increase the weight by 1–2 pounds every workout until you reach a four again.

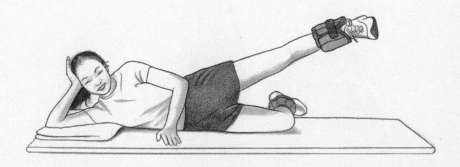

HIP ADDUCTION ◆

This exercise will strengthen the muscles on the inside of the thigh. These muscles are used when you get out of a chair, climb, or move from side to side as you do when you play tennis or other sports. They also provide balance in the case of stumbling.

Starting position: Lie on the floor on your back with your knees bent. One leg at a time, raise your legs so they are extended perpendicular to the floor, with the bottom of your feet facing the ceiling.

1-2-3-Down: Open your legs simultaneously to form a "V." Open your legs as wide as is comfortable without arching your back or letting your legs drift toward your head or the ground.

Pause for 1 second.

1-2-Up: Squeeze your legs together to close the "V," again without letting them drift toward your head or the ground.

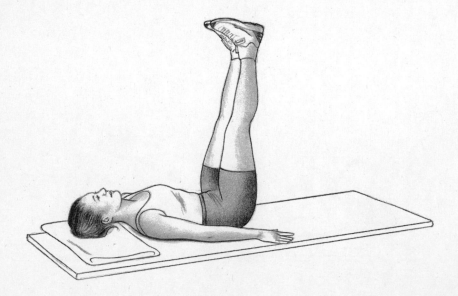

Reps and sets: Repeat the move until you have done 12 repetitions—this is 1 set. Rest for about 30 seconds and then do a second set.

Focal points: Relax your upper body during the movement. Do not tense your shoulders or neck muscles. Keep the bottoms of your feet facing up toward the ceiling. With your lower legs relaxed, initiate the movement from the inner thighs and visualize the inner thighs contracting. Be aware of overstretching the inner thigh. Only open the "V" as wide as is comfortable—you don't want to pull a muscle.

Progressions

1. Most people's inner thigh muscles are notoriously weak. If you can't get down on the floor and lift your legs into the up position, start by lying on the floor with your knees bent and putting two pillows or a tennis ball between your legs and squeeze. Hold the squeeze 5–10 seconds. Perform 12 repetitions. Once your inner thighs and trunk muscles become stronger, you can do this exercise as described above.

2. Start by only lowering your legs a few inches once they are in the "up" position.

3. As you become stronger, lower your legs as far as possible.

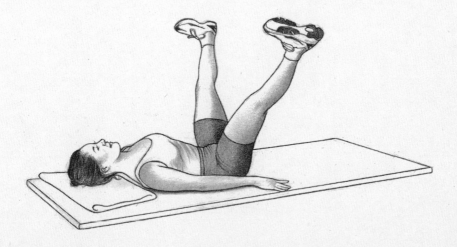

Stage 2 for Hip Osteoarthritis: Weeks 5–8

Back extension: See pages 108–109.

Modified boat pose: See pages 110–111.

Stage 3 for Hip Osteoarthritis: Weeks 9–12

Lateral shoulder raise: See pages 119–121.

Reverse fly: See pages 116–118.

Stage 4 for Hip Osteoarthritis: Weeks 13–16

Try the squat or step-up (pages 99–103), and see if you can do either or both without significant pain. If so, add them to your program. If they are still painful, continue with what you have been doing, and every couple of weeks attempt the squat and step-up again.

ARTHRITIS OF THE HANDS, WRISTS, OR ELBOWS

If you have arthritis of the hands, wrists, or elbows, add these two exercises to the basic program. Remember that if you have difficulty gripping the dumbbells, you can buy adjustable wrist weights that fit snugly around your wrists. *Note:* Flexibility exercises have also been shown to be beneficial for osteoarthritis of the hand and will be outlined in the "Flexibility" section (page 135).

Wrist extension and flexion

These two exercises will strengthen the forearm muscles. Strength in these muscles will improve your grip strength. It is helpful for those with arthritis in the hands and/or wrists.

If you have rheumatoid or another inflammatory arthritis of the hands and wrists, pay special attention to how these joints feel the morning after this exercise. If you have more or longer pain and stiffness than before, cut down to 8 repetitions until you are able to do this without pain or added stiffness.

WRIST EXTENSION ◆

Starting position: Sit in a chair with a table on your right side. With good posture, keep your hips all the way back in the chair with your feet flat on the floor, hip-width apart. Holding a small weight in your hand, rest your right forearm on the table, palm facing down. Your wrist should extend just past the edge of the table.

1-2-Up: Lift your hand up and back toward your trunk by cocking your wrist up while keeping your forearm down on the table. Your forearm will be supported by the table.

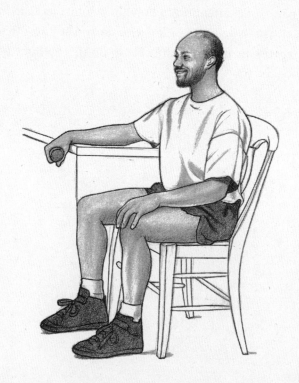

Pause for 1 second at the top of the movement.

1-2-3-Down: Lower your hand to the starting position.

Reps and sets: Do 12 repetitions on one side, rest, and repeat. Then turn the chair around so the table is on the left side, and repeat the move for the left arm.

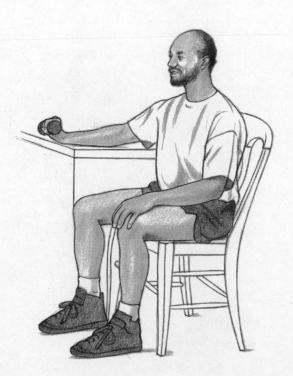

WRIST FLEXION ◆

Starting position: This requires the same position as the extension, except your forearm will rest on the table with the palm facing *up*.

1-2-Up: Lift your hand up and back toward your trunk, keeping your forearm on the table. The table will support your forearm.

Pause for 1 second at the top of the movement.

1-2-3-Down: Lower your hand to the starting position.

Reps and sets: Do 12 repetitions on one side, rest, and repeat. Then turn the chair around so the table is on the left side, and repeat the move for the left arm.

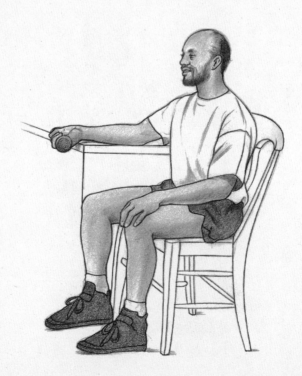

Focal points for both wrist exercises: Keep both sides of your forearm down during the movement. Lift and lower in the greatest range of motion you can manage while still performing the exercise correctly and pain free.

Progressions (for both extension and flexion)
1. Start without any weight until you can do 12 repetitions in good form and the intensity is less than a four on the intensity scale.
2. Progress to holding a 1-pound weight in each hand. As you become stronger and the intensity drops below a four on the intensity scale, increase the weight in each hand by 1-pound increments each workout until you reach a four on the intensity scale.

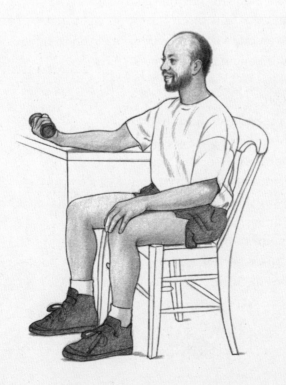

Handgrips for grip strength

There are a number of different devices available to help strengthen your grip. We recommend you try some of them. Have them available on the coffee table to use while you read or watch TV or if you are a passenger in a car, train, or plane. There are two basic types of devices available to strengthen your hand and forearm. The first category includes foam or neoprene handgrips. These focus primarily on forearm strength but work the fingers as well. The handgrip consists of two handles connected by a high-tension spring, which provides resistance. Both handles fit in the palm of your hand, and you squeeze them. The other category is comprised of squeeze balls, which are exactly that—balls that fit in your hand and provide resistance when you squeeze them. They come in different resistances, with some more difficult to squeeze than others. Decide on the appropriate resistance before you buy one. You can always increase the resistance as you get stronger. The handgrips are around three dollars, and the balls run from five to eight dollars. Many brands come with descriptions of exercises you can do with the devices. They are available at most sporting goods stores.

Squeeze Ball

Grip the squeeze ball in your hand and slowly squeeze the ball as hard as you can for 5–10 seconds, then relax. Repeat the sequence five times and then switch to the other hand for 5 repetitions. Increase the intensity of the move by squeezing the ball up to 30 seconds for each repetition. During the 30 seconds, squeeze each finger particularly hard for 6 seconds.

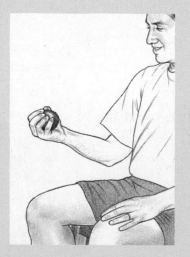

FLEXIBILITY: GENERAL GUIDELINES

The components of a joint's flexibility, or range of motion, include three things: the elasticity of connective tissues in the joint, muscle tension, and strength. Strength training covers strength, of course. The flexibility exercises here will target elasticity of the connective tissue (tendons and ligaments) and muscle tension.

Just as the goal of strength training is to "overload" the muscle in order for it to adapt and get stronger, the goal with flexibility is to "overstretch." That is, in order to develop flexibility, your current range of motion must be exceeded. However, flexibility training stresses muscles in a different way from strengthening, in that it does not require the day of rest between sessions for positive adaptation to occur. In fact, the greatest increases in flexibility come with stretching every day.

It takes time to develop flexibility, and progress is measured in quarter-inch and half-inch increments, so it is important to set realistic goals and reward yourself for small gains. These small gains will eventually turn into larger ones and reap many benefits, such as fewer aches and pains, greater range of motion (and therefore freedom of movement), and less chance of injury.

As you do these exercises, don't compare yourself to others. Flexibility varies from person to person. The point is for you to become more flexible than you were at the start—not as flexible or more flexible than someone else.

How to do the exercises

It is very important to warm up before stretching in order to increase muscle temperature and the flow of fluid into the joints. That will promote more effective stretching and decrease the risk of injury. Because you will do your stretching at the end of your workout, you will be sufficiently warmed up, either from strength training or aerobic exercise. Each stretch will be performed twice.

As we discussed, you must stretch *beyond* your current comfortable range of motion in order to improve flexibility. Thus, the amount you stretch may produce some discomfort at first, especially for beginners, but never to the point of being painful. Because discomfort and pain are subjective matters, you must use common sense. But if your muscle quivers, if pain persists, or if your range of motion *decreases,* you have stretched too much.

The movement in the exercise should be slow and deliberate, and then static (unmoving) for a period of time when you reach your endpoint, which is the point that it feels tight but is not painful. Work to hold the stretch at the endpoint for 30 seconds. This will produce the greatest gain in flexibility, but 15 seconds will also bring some improvement. We will start with 15 seconds and, over the weeks, work up to 30 seconds. Do not hesitate to hold the stretch for longer than 30 seconds if it feels good and you feel the tightness letting go, but shoot for a minimum of 30 seconds over time. And always remember to breathe throughout the stretch.

For stretching to be most beneficial, *make sure your form is correct.* For example, when you stretch the back of the thighs in the hamstring stretch described on page 138, if you round your back you will be overstretching your lower back. You will also be compressing your spine and not properly focusing on your hamstrings.

LUNGE STRETCH ◆

Stand with good posture next to a sturdy table. Take a step forward with
your right leg so that your feet are about 4 feet apart. Your right foot will
be directly in front of your left foot. Place your right hand on the table to
steady your balance. Keep your trunk and head centered over your hips. Do
not lean forward or back. Take in a breath, and on the exhalation bend your
right leg until you feel a stretch in the front of your left hip and/or left calf.
You may have to lift your left heel off the floor if your calf is tight. Your goal
is to eventually keep that heel on the floor with a considerable bend (close to
90 degrees) in your right knee. Keep your right knee directly over your ankle,
adjusting the distance between your feet if you need to. Use your hands on
your hips to check that your hips are level and square. The back leg should
be strong and straight. If you feel off balance, move your left leg out slightly
to widen your base of support. Once you are in the stretch, relax the upper
body and breath into the tight muscle. Hold the stretch for 15 seconds and
then repeat. Switch legs and repeat the stretch 2 times for 15 seconds on the
other side. After 4 weeks, increase the time to 30 seconds for each stretch.

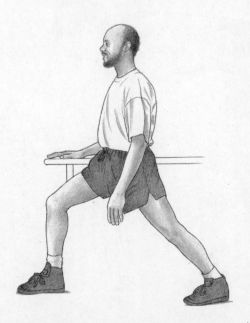

HAMSTRING STRETCH ◆

Stand with your feet hip-width apart, knees slightly bent. Do not lock your knees. Pull your tailbone underneath you slightly. Bend forward from the hips, and place your outstretched hands on a chair (or table if the chair is too low). Keep your neck in line with your spine, keeping your entire back straight. Center your hips over your ankles. You will feel a stronger stretch in the back of the thighs when you do this. Only go as far as you can while maintaining good posture—do not round your back. You will benefit much more by doing the stretch properly but not going down too far, and you will avoid injuring your back. Repeat the stretch twice for 15 seconds. After 4 weeks, increase the time to 30 seconds.

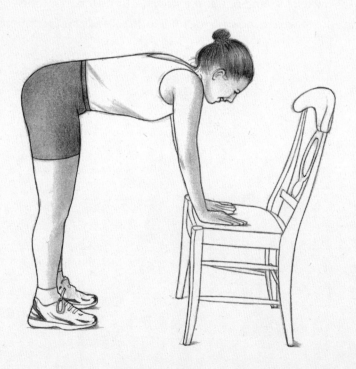

CROSSOVER FOR BUTTOCKS AND HIPS ◆

Lie on your back on the floor with your legs extended. Stretch out your left arm in line with your shoulder. Grasp the outside of your left knee or thigh with your right hand. Inhale, and then as you exhale pull your left knee across your body toward the floor. Keep your shoulders and head on the floor. Pull your left leg across your body until you feel the stretch in the outside of your left hip. You may also feel it on the left side of your trunk. Do the same stretch on your right side for the right hip and buttock. Perform the stretch twice for 15 seconds on both sides. After 4 weeks, increase the time to 30 seconds for each stretch.

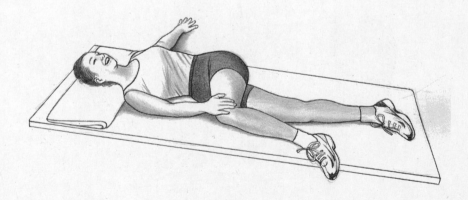

QUADRICEPS STRETCH ◆

Level 1: Stand to the side of a chair. Bend your left knee, bring your heel toward your buttocks, and rest your foot on the chair—your left knee will form a right angle. Keep the knee of your right leg slightly bent throughout the move to avoid straining it as your right leg supports your weight. Breathe through the stretch.

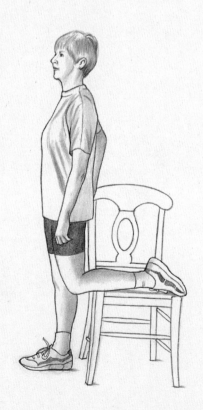

Level 2: Stand behind a chair. Bend your left knee, bring your heel toward your buttocks, and grasp your foot with your left hand. Pull the heel toward your buttocks. Do not arch your lower back to get the heel closer. Keep your knee in line with your hip: Do not pull it out, in, forward, or back. As with level 1, keep the knee of your right leg bent slightly throughout the move to avoid straining it.

For Levels 1 and 2: Perform the stretch twice for 15 seconds on both sides. After 4 weeks, increase the time to 30 seconds for each stretch.

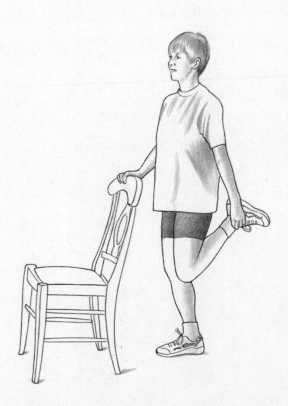

SHOULDER STRETCH ◆

Stand with your feet hip-width apart, knees slightly bent. Relax your shoulders down and back, and keep your head in line with your spine. Interlock your fingers, turn your palms out, and stretch your arms forward. (If you can't turn your wrists enough to interlock your fingers, bend your wrists back as far as they will go and touch the fingertips of the two hands together.) Lift them up toward your head, keeping your shoulders down

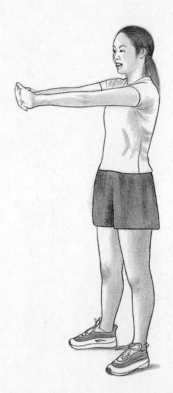

and back. Keep raising your arms until you feel a stretch in the shoulders. As you lift, do not arch your lower back or drop your head forward. Relax and breathe throughout the stretch. The maximum endpoint is reached when your arms are straight above your shoulders, elbows next to your ears. Keep turning your palms away from you. You will also feel this stretch in the forearms. It does not matter how far you raise your arms, just that the posture is correct and you feel a stretch. Perform the stretch twice for 15 seconds each time. After 4 weeks, increase the time to 30 seconds.

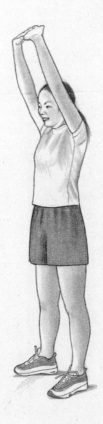

WRIST STRETCHES ◆

These two stretches will improve the flexibility of the wrists and fingers.
Stand facing a table. Put your arms straight down with hands on the table,
palms down with fingers facing toward your legs and spread out. Inhale,
and then as you exhale lean back until you feel a stretch in your forearms,
wrists, and palms.

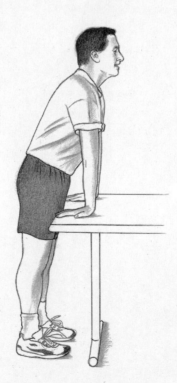

Now, put your arms straight down with palms up (do not lock elbows; keep them soft) and fingers facing back and spread out. Inhale, and as you exhale lean back until you feel the stretch in the forearms and wrists.

Perform each move twice for 15 seconds. After 4 weeks, increase the time to 30 seconds.

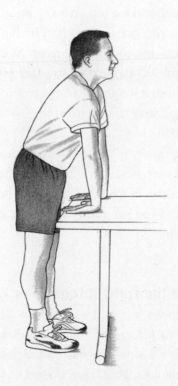

AEROBIC EXERCISE: GENERAL GUIDELINES

Aerobic activity can be weight bearing or non–weight bearing. "Weight bearing" means that while you do the exercise, you are holding up the weight of your body on your legs. Brisk walking is a weight-bearing aerobic activity. Bicycle riding is non–weight bearing—the seat of the bike is bearing much of your weight.

We recommend doing weight-bearing exercise or a combination of weight-bearing and non-weight-bearing aerobic exercise. Weight-bearing activity has been shown to be vital to maintaining cartilage integrity.

Examples of weight-bearing and non-weight-bearing exercises and guidelines for performing them will be provided at the end of this section. The activity you choose will depend, in part, on what you can do pain free. If higher-impact, weight-bearing aerobic exercises like walking and aerobics classes are too painful, try weight-bearing activities with less impact, such as cross-country skiing and working out on an elliptical trainer. If these fail, engage in non-weight-bearing exercises such as biking, swimming, or rowing. Wherever you start from, always try to progress to some weight-bearing exercise as you go forward. As you become stronger with the strength-training program, you may find that weight-bearing aerobic activities get easier. Increasing muscle strength may take some of the load off your joints or more evenly distribute the load.

The key to getting results from aerobic exercise, just as with strength-training and flexibility exercises, is to work out at the right level of intensity. There is a range you want to work in: Too low and you will see little improvement; too high and you risk injury as well as no improvement because of overtaxing the system.

How to determine the right intensity or range

The range you want to work in is described as a percentage of your maximum heart rate: 60–80 percent of maximum heart rate is the desirable range. This is safely within your capability but high enough to give your cardiovascular system a good workout. How do you know your maximum heart rate—and how do you know when you are between 60 and 80 percent of that? First, maximum heart rate is exactly that—the maximum attainable rate your heart can beat. It is predicted by a simple equation:

MAXIMUM HEART RATE = 220 minus your age in years

Age is factored into the equation because there are changes in the pumping of the heart as we get older. It is important to note that there is considerable variability from person to person in this predicted maximum heart rate, so *use it as a ballpark measure* in conjunction with how you feel, not as an absolute number.

Once you know your maximum heart rate, there are two ways to gauge 60–80 percent of that. One is to take your pulse during exercise. The other involves the use of an intensity scale. If you are a new exerciser and are unfamiliar with the feeling of aerobic exertion, we recommend that you use the pulse method at first to become familiar with the way it feels to train at 60, 70, and 80 percent of your maximum heart rate. After you become familiar with this feeling, use the intensity scale, or a combination of pulse rate and intensity scale.

Learning your target heart rate

To find out what 60–80 percent of your maximum is, you can multiply your maximum heart rate by 0.60 and 0.80 to get 60 and 80 percent, respectively. Or you can use the chart on the next page, where the math has been done for you. For each age, the maximum heart rate has already been calculated, and the chart provides the percentages of this maximum.

TARGET HEART RATE = 60–80 percent of MAXIMUM HEART RATE

Once you know what your heart rate should be, you need to know how to measure it by taking your pulse during your aerobic training. To take your pulse: Hold your right hand out. Press together the index finger and middle finger of your left hand and touch them to the base of your right thumb on the inside of your wrist. Slide the fingers across your wrist, moving them parallel to the top of your right arm. Press firmly when you're at the hollow next to the tendons. You should be able to feel your pulse. If not, vary how firmly you are pressing. It may also help to bend your right wrist back

	HEART RATE IN BEATS PER MINUTE AT DIFFERENT PERCENTS OF MAXIMUM			
AGE	60%	70%	80%	90%
20	120	140	160	180
25	117	137	156	176
30	114	133	152	171
35	111	130	148	167
40	108	126	144	162
45	105	123	140	158
50	102	119	136	153
55	99	116	132	149
60	96	112	128	144
65	93	109	124	140
70	90	105	120	135
75	87	102	116	131
80	84	98	112	126

slightly. Watching the clock, count the number of beats in a given period of time (see below). To determine your pulse rate, multiply the number of pulses you get by the number of counting intervals in 1 minute to get beats per minute. The longer you count your pulse, the more accurate it will be. There can be as much as a one-beat error during the count, and this error is magnified when you count for a shorter period of time.

- If you count for 15 seconds, multiply by 4 to get beats per minute.
- If you count for 20 seconds, multiply by 3 to get beats per minute.
- If you count for 30 seconds, multiply by 2 to get beats per minute.

Check your heart rate when you're 5 minutes into aerobic activity and at the end, just before you cool down. That way, you can tell whether you're pushing yourself hard enough (at least 60 percent of your maximum heart rate) but not too much (more than 80 percent). Of course, you can also check it whenever you want to know how hard you're working.

Caution: Don't take your pulse at your neck. You'll be pressing on your carotid artery, which could impede blood flow to your brain.

You don't have to use your fingers to take your pulse. You can also measure your heart rate with a heart rate monitor. Heart rate monitors can be purchased at sporting goods stores, ranging in price from $50–$200. A strap is worn around your mid-chest in conjunction with a watch that is worn on your wrist. Transmitters on the chest strap send a signal to the watch, which receives the signal and reads out your heart rate.

Intensity scale

Once you have determined what the proper intensity feels like by matching your target pulse rate during aerobic exercise to how your body responds (a certain amount of sweating, heavy breathing, etc.), you're ready to use an intensity scale to determine whether you're working out between 60 and 80 percent of your maximum heart rate. The scale is a 5-point scale, similar to what you used in the strength program, but the levels correspond with your heart rate versus how fatigued your muscles feel. Level 3 corresponds with 60–80 percent of heart rate maximum.

The talk test is one way of using the scale to determine the intensity of your exercise. Generally, exercising above 90 percent of your maximum heart rate does not allow you to utter more than a word or two at a time. The ability to talk with frequent interruptions for breathing corresponds with a four on the intensity scale. You should be able to continue talking when you are working out at an intensity of three.

Caution for measuring intensity

If you have a cardiac pacemaker or are taking medications that can raise or lower your heart rate—including cold remedies, appetite suppressants, beta blockers or calcium channel blockers for high blood pressure—discuss exer-

EXERCISE INTENSITY SCALE
FOR AEROBIC TRAINING

Exercise intensity level	Description of effort
1. Sedentary	No perceived effort: standing, sitting, or lying down.
2. Active This level contributes to overall health and burns more calories than being sedentary.	Easy, sustainable movement that causes a small increase in heart and breathing rate and doesn't raise a sweat (unless the weather is hot): strolling, gardening, slow dancing, golfing.
3. Aerobic training You should exercise at this level to condition your heart and lungs.	Somewhat hard movement that elevates the heart rate to 60–70 percent of maximum most of the time, ranging up to 80 percent. Breathing is more rapid, though it's possible to converse with only slightly altered speech; perspiration appears after about 5–15 minutes, depending on air temperature.
4. Athletic training This is a more advanced level of aerobic conditioning that might become an appropriate goal after the 16-week program.	Hard effort that elevates the heart rate to 70–80 percent most of the time, ranging up to 90 percent of maximum. Breathing is more rapid but not labored—it's possible to converse, though faster breathing will cause evident interruptions; perspiration will start within 5–10 minutes, depending on air temperature; fatigue will increase as the workout continues, and you will feel a need to stop by the end.
5. Overexertion Not recommended!	Excessive effort: heart pounds to the point of discomfort or nausea; breathing is too rapid to permit speech.

cise intensity goals with your doctor before you start. These medications affect your heart rate, which will render inaccurate the reading you get by taking your pulse or using the intensity scale. It is also important to note environmental conditions that can affect your heart rate. For example, in hot, humid environments, the body has a harder time getting rid of its heat, so working out at the same intensity may result in heart rates 10–20 beats higher per minute than usual. Be thoughtful when measuring your intensity, and go by how you feel as well as your heart rate.

How to start

If you have not been doing any aerobic exercises, we recommend starting with 5–10 minutes of an activity at a low intensity. Just do it, as they say—do not worry about intensity or effort. Spending the first 2 weeks simply getting used to doing aerobic activity is a great way to start. Afterward, you can begin to increase the length of time and intensity as outlined below. As with the strength-training program, you will start out slowly and progress over the first weeks to the desired intensity—60–80 percent of heart rate maximum. As you become more fit, you will find you will have to increase the intensity of your workout to keep your heart rate in this range.

If you have been doing some sort of aerobic exercise but not monitoring intensity, begin by monitoring your heart rate or intensity, and over the first three weeks work up to the appropriate intensity as outlined below.

Frequency
Perform aerobic exercise three times a week. You may do it on consecutive days if you like—you don't have to skip a day between aerobic workouts.

Week 1	40–50% HR max	5–10 minutes
Week 2	50% HR max	10 minutes
Week 3	60% HR max	15 minutes
Week 4	60–70% HR max	15 minutes
Week 5 and beyond	60–80% HR max	20 minutes

Maintain the 20 minutes at 60–80 percent three times a week.

Warm up and cool down
The best warm-up and cool-down activity is the same one you plan to do at your target heart rate, only at a lower intensity. Always start your aerobic

workout slowly, and take 5 minutes to work up to your target heart rate. It is important to warm up your muscles before you take them through more strenuous exercise. Cooling down is just as important to gradually ease the muscles out of the more strenuous work. Simply do the warm-up in reverse: Spend 5 minutes slowing down your activity at the end of the workout. You need not add extra time onto your workout to warm up and cool down. Make it part of the time you are exercising. So when you are exercising for 20 minutes at a time by 5 weeks, you will be in your target heart rate for 10 minutes and gradually building up to it and coming down from it for the other 10 minutes. At the beginning, when you are exercising for shorter periods of time, decrease the warm-up and cool-down time to only a couple minutes for each.

Types of activities

The most important thing about the activity you choose is that you like doing it. For instance, if you hate to walk or it is painful to walk, it is unlikely that you will maintain a walking program.

Weight-bearing aerobic exercises

WALKING/HIKING: This is probably the easiest activity because it is readily available to most people. It can be done just about anywhere with limited equipment—just a good pair of shoes (not worn out). Remember, however, that walking for aerobic exercise does not mean strolling as you gab with a friend, or window shopping, but instead walking briskly so that your body becomes warm (and you eventually break into a sweat) and you feel your heart rate rise. Besides increasing your speed in order to work up a sweat, you can raise the intensity of a walking workout by taking a hike on hilly terrain—a great activity to plan for longer workouts on the weekends. Treadmill walking can be lower in impact than walking outdoors—good for people whose knees really crunch. The surface on the treadmill has more give. Treadmills also allow you to control the speed and incline in order to vary your workout.

CROSS-COUNTRY SKI MACHINES AND ELLIPTICAL TRAINERS: Although the exercises performed on these machines are weight bearing, they don't create as much force on the skeleton as exercises in which your foot actually hits the ground. That can be an important advantage, because their gliding movements are easier on the joints. Actual cross-country skiing as well as snow-shoeing are great outdoor winter workouts. Like the machines, they're weight bearing but allow for low impact on the joints.

STAIR-STEPPING MACHINES: These should be used with caution. They can put undue stress on the joints if care is not taken to perform the stepping properly. Follow the guidelines for stepping as described in the step-up exercise on page 102–103.

EXERCISE CLASSES: These can range from low-impact aerobics classes to boxing to dancing. There are many low-impact options that will decrease stress on the joints. Most exercise classes improve coordination and balance, too. Instructors usually include a warm-up, cool-down, and stretch. Before you select a class, read a description or, better yet, talk with the instructor to learn if the required fitness level and type of exercise are appropriate for you.

If going to a class is not for you because you prefer exercising solo in the privacy of your own home, you can bring some of the fun of an aerobics class into your home with exercise videos. If possible, rent a video before you buy it to make sure it's appropriate and enjoyable.

Non-weight-bearing aerobic exercises

BIKING: Many people with osteoarthritis of the knee who find weight-bearing activities too painful at first can start with biking. You can cycle around town on your own bike or use a stationary bike—or a combination. If you are riding your own bike, make sure that you are fit enough to be safe and steady and that the bike fits you. If you use a stationary bike, it can be upright or "recumbent" (meaning that you semi-recline as you cycle). Those with back problems sometimes find the recumbent bikes less stressful on their spines. You can also get stands to prop up your own bike indoors and ride it like a stationary bike.

ROWING: Rowing is a great whole-body aerobic exercise. Just make sure that you get proper instruction, as rowing can be hard on the knee joints if you perform the move improperly.

SWIMMING: This is probably the best non-weight-bearing, whole-body exercise for people with arthritis. Water activities are very soothing for individuals with arthritis, as the water helps to unload body weight from the painful joints. There are now so many more options than just swimming laps. You can take water aerobics classes or walk or run in the water for a low-impact workout. Even if you can't swim, all you have to do is get in the water to mid-chest depth and walk. The resistance of the water will make it hard to move so that you can increase your heart rate without having to run. Equipment available for walking or jogging in the water includes a buoyancy belt, which keeps your head above water for deep-water running. There are also flippers and dumbbells that can be used while you are running or walking in deep water to increase resistance and, therefore, the intensity of the workout.

GOOD PAIN AND BAD PAIN

Pain doesn't only hurt. It can be scary because it might seem like a sign that you have injured yourself. But when you begin an exercise program—or return to one after many years—you are bound to feel some pain or achiness, at least at first. In fact, you're *supposed* to feel some soreness. It means you're challenging your muscles and that they are responding and getting stronger. But you need to know the difference between the "good" pain that tells you you're doing things right and the "bad" pain that could signal that you've overdone it or are moving your body incorrectly and need to take a break. How can you tell which is which?

If you feel fine during an exercise session itself but experience muscle aches the next day, that's good pain. Called *delayed muscle soreness,* it's caused by what are known as eccentric muscle contractions—the part of the lift when you lower the weight or, in aerobic exercise, the impact on muscles as they lengthen. Either way, you may feel a general achiness all over, as if you were coming down with the flu. That's okay, too. The muscle soreness is generally pretty mild and will go away on its own within a couple of days.

Do *not* take painkillers or increase your dose of pain medication to relieve the discomfort. That can interfere with the body's natural mechanism for repairing the microscopic muscle tears that cause the soreness. Also, if you use painkillers to deal with pain from routine exercise, you won't be able to "hear" signals from your body about whether you're pushing yourself too hard (a possibility if you start out extremely enthusiastic but out of shape). Better to relieve your muscles by stretching them with some of the flexibility exercises. Soaking in a hot bath might also relax your muscles, as will massaging the ones you can reach.

After a couple of weeks, good pain should manifest itself as nothing more than muscle fatigue right after you finish a strength-training set or aerobic activity. It comes from the burning of lactic acid, which is the muscles' normal response to working hard. The fatigue, or burn, should dissipate within minutes.

Bad pain, a sign that you need to back off, is not dull. It's sharp. It generally doesn't mean you've done severe damage to yourself, but it does mean you need to give your body a break and reexamine your routine.

Do not start exercising again until the sharp pain disappears. If things are going too slowly, try speeding them along by elevating the joint and applying ice to it. But if the pain is severe—or gets worse—see your doctor.

When you do start exercising again, drop down one progression in strength training from where you were, just to play it safe, or decrease the intensity of your aerobic workout. And have a friend or family member watch you, or look in the mirror, to make sure you're doing the strength-training movements properly. If all goes well, you can step up the progression after two sessions. But if the sharp pain reappears, seek medical attention.

If you have rheumatoid arthritis and experience a flare-up, that's a time to step back at least one progression in strength training and decrease the duration and intensity of aerobic activities to an amount that you can comfortably tolerate. During flare-ups you *are* encouraged to continue doing your flexibility exercises. The stretching will relieve some of the aches, pains, and muscle tension. Once the flare-ups subside, you can resume your normal routine.

Rest assured that most people who use our program do not experience bad pain. Because our program starts out slowly and builds up gradually, we see very few injuries in the arthritis patients we work with. But if you do end up with any sharp pain, do not let it discourage you. If you work with our suggestions, you will generally be able to overcome these small, albeit uncomfortable, obstacles. Remember, we all run up against challenges. It's how we address those challenges that determines the outcome.

Snap, crackle, pop

Many of our research volunteers ask us about noises that come from their knee joint when they exercise. They wonder whether they should be concerned. As long as the sounds are not accompanied by sharp pain, the answer is no. The noises are caused simply by irregularities of the cartilage underneath the kneecap. They can also be caused by a group of inflammatory cells on the lining of the tendon called *nodules.* The sounds, or "pops," are more common in women than in men.

PLANNING YOUR WORKOUTS FOR THE FIRST SIXTEEN WEEKS

Plan your workout according to what fits your schedule and will keep you most motivated. Be realistic. Some people prefer to work out for a shorter period over more days, while others prefer to do a few longer workouts. Below are two possibilities that suit these two types: a 3-day plan and a 6-day plan. These are certainly not the only options. You may start with these and, as you become familiar with the exercises, create your own individualized program. Just remember to allow a day's rest before strength training the same muscle group again. Remember, too, that the most important part of your exercise program is making it a way of life. So create a program that works for you; that you will stick with; and that you'll modify when you need to.

A three-day option

For this option you will do all the components of the program on 1 day: aerobic, strength training, and stretching. At the beginning, the program will take you about 20 minutes. By the end of 16 weeks, the entire program will take you 1 hour 15 minutes. You will warm up for strength training by doing the aerobic program and cool down from your entire workout by stretching at the end.

A six-day option

Three days a week during the 6-day option you will do strength training and stretching, and on the alternate days you will do aerobic exercise and stretching. The aerobic workouts will last about 30 minutes, and the strength training, once you have added all the exercises at week 13, will take just under 1 hour. The stretching will take about 5 minutes.

PROGRAM SUMMARY

The table on the following page contains a summary of the program, showing when each exercise is introduced during each of the four stages as well as indicating the progressions for the aerobic exercise portion of the program. You decide for yourself whether to do all the exercises in 3 days a week or to spread them out over 6 days.

WHAT'S NEXT?

When the same stimulus is repeated over and over, the body will adapt by making fewer and fewer improvements, and you will go for a period of time without making any significant gains. This plateau in your training is okay if you are happy with your achievements and would just like to maintain them. As we discussed earlier in the chapter, it is by stressing the system via overloading or overstretching, and by allowing proper recovery after exercising, that the body will become more fit than it was before you started exercising.

However, you may become mentally and physically "stale" with the same exercises and with repeating the same routine over and over, which makes it difficult to sustain enough intensity even for the maintenance of your new gains. If you're bored, you're more apt to do the exercises with less enthusiasm.

EXERCISE	STAGE 1 *Weeks 1–4*	STAGE 2 *Weeks 5–8*	STAGE 3 *Weeks 9–12*	STAGE 4 *Weeks 13–16*
Aerobic exercise	3 × week	3 × week	3 × week	3 × week
Duration	5–15 minutes	20 minutes	20 minutes	20 minutes
Intensity scale	Levels 2–3	Level 3	Level 3	Level 3
Strength training (2 sets of 12 reps)	3 × week	3 × week	3 × week	3 × week
Modified squat	×	×	×	×
Step-up	×	×	×	×
Toe stands	×	×	×	×
Modified push-up	×	×	×	×
*Back extension		×	×	×
*Modified boat pose		×	×	×
Knee extension			×	×
Knee flexion			×	×
Reverse fly				×
Lateral shoulder raises				×
Stretches (2 × 30 seconds each)	After exercise	After exercise	After exercise	After exercise
Lunge				
Hamstring				
Crossover				
Quadriceps				
Shoulder stretch				
Wrist stretch (optional)				

*Only complete 5 repetitions for the back extension and modified boat pose.

In order to continue seeing results over the long term—for months and years—it is important to vary the intensity, frequency, and/or type of exercises you are doing. This will keep your body on its toes with new stimuli to adapt to as well as keep you fresh mentally. Consider the following options for the three types of exercises we recommend in our program.

Strength-training variations

After you have completed the 16-week program, maintain Stage 4 for another 4 weeks. After that, *decrease* the intensity to a three (by dropping down a progression) and do more repetitions to fatigue (15 repetitions). Continue this for a week and then dive back into the higher intensity. Cycling these periods of lower intensity (1 week) with high intensity (8 weeks) will prevent overloading the muscles too much and also stave off mental fatigue. Remember, it is a balance of rest and work that will yield the greatest improvements.

You can also "mix things up" by switching some of the exercises you are doing every 8 weeks. Replace one upper-body and one lower-body exercise with new ones that target the same muscles. Your muscles can become adapted to the same motion or exercise, and you may begin to plateau. The new exercises will nudge you forward again. Below are suggestions for new exercises and what they replace.

STATIONARY LUNGE
(Replaces the Step-Up) ◆

This exercise will strengthen the front of the thighs and the backs of the legs and hips.

Starting position: Stand next to a table or counter with the right foot 3–4 feet in front of the left foot and hip-width apart, knees slightly bent. Focus on something at eye level. Gently hold onto the counter or table for balance.

1-2-3-Down: Keeping your upper body erect, drop your hips straight down and bend both knees. The heel of your back leg will come off the floor as you bend down. Your front leg will be close to parallel to the floor, and your back knee will be several inches off the floor.

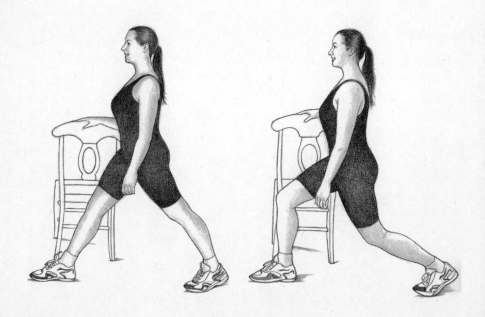

Pause for 1 second.

1-2-Up: Push through both legs to return to the starting position.

Reps and sets: Repeat the move 12 times with the right leg forward, then switch legs and perform the move another 12 times with the left leg forward—this is 1 set. Rest for about 30 seconds and then do a second set.

Focal points: Do not use the table to support your weight by leaning on it. Use it only for balance. Maintain posture in the upper body as you descend and ascend, keeping your shoulders and head in line with your hips. Keep the forward leg over the ankle (not in front of it) and in line with the toes. Depending on how tall you are, you may need to adjust the distance between your feet. Distribute your weight between the balls and heels of your feet and equally between the front and back leg.

Progressions
1. Use the counter for balance and lower with both knees. If you cannot maintain good form when you rise up, decrease the depth of your descent. Increase the intensity as you get stronger by dropping down further toward the floor and by spreading the distance between your legs. Work toward getting your front thigh parallel to the floor.
2. When the intensity drops below a four, increase the intensity by not using the counter or table for balance.
3. When you can perform the exercise in the full range of motion without using your hand for balance and the intensity drops below a four, hold a 5-pound dumbbell in each hand while you do the exercise. Progress to 8 pounds, 10 pounds, and 12 pounds as you get stronger.

WALL SLIDE (Replaces the Modified Squat) ◆

This exercise strengthens the fronts and backs of the thighs and can be done anywhere.

Starting position: Lean your back against a wall with your feet approximately 2 feet out in front of you (a little more if you have long legs) and your knees slightly bent. Focus on something at eye level. Feet should be hip-width apart and parallel.

1-2-3-Down: Bend your knees slightly, and pull your tailbone down slightly so that you feel the back of your waist come in contact with the wall. Lower yourself down the wall, keeping your knees over your ankles and in line with your toes. You may have to adjust the distance of your feet from the wall to maintain the knee-over-ankle position.

Lower to the distance at which you feel you can hold the position for several breaths (about 5 seconds).

1-2-Up: Return to the starting position by sliding back up the wall.

Repeat the move a total of 5 times.

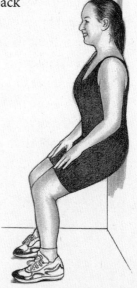

Focal points: Keep your back against the wall and your head in line with your spine. Relax your neck, shoulders, and arms. Breathe, releasing any tension in your upper body as you hold the sitting position.

Progressions

1. Increase the amount of time you hold the position to 10 seconds, then 15 and 20 seconds.

2. Once you can hold the position 5 times for 20 seconds, increase the descent down the wall so that your knees form a right angle.

CHEST FLY (Replaces the Wall Push-ups) ◆

This exercise strengthens the chest and front shoulders.

Starting position: Lie on your back on the floor with your knees bent and feet flat on the floor, hip-width apart. Place your arms out to your sides at shoulder height with palms facing up. Elbows should be slightly bent.

1-2-Up: Bring your arms together over your chest in an arcing motion. Your elbows will remain soft but fixed in the starting position as you lift. During the motion, do not let your arms drift forward or back.

Pause for 1 second when your hands or the weights in your hands almost touch.

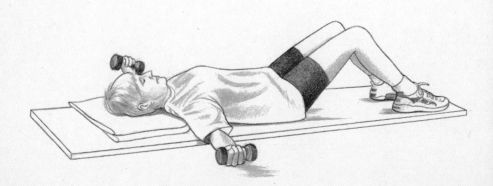

1-2-3-Down: Lower your arms to the starting position in the same motion.

Reps and sets: Repeat the move until you have done 12 repetitions— this is 1 set. Rest for about 30 seconds and then do a second set.

Focal points: Do not lift your hips or arch your back during the movement. Initiate the movement from the shoulders and chest, not the elbows. Visualize your chest muscles squeezing together. When holding the weight, keep your wrist neutral. Avoid letting the weight bring the wrist into extension or flexion.

Progressions

1. Practice the exercise without weight until you can do 12 repetitions in good form. Then start with a 1- to 3-pound weight in each hand and increase the weight by 1 pound per workout until the intensity is a four on the scale after 2 sets of 12 repetitions.

2. As you become stronger and the intensity decreases below a four, increase the weight of the dumbbells by 1- to 3-pound increments per workout to reach a four on the intensity scale.

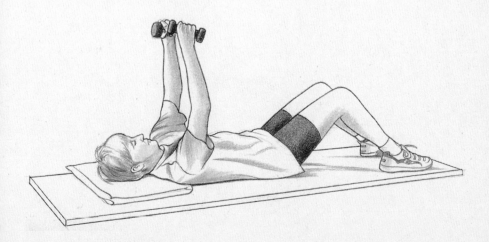

OVERHEAD PRESS (Replaces the Lateral Shoulder Raise) ◆

This exercise will strengthen the shoulder muscles, especially those of the front and middle shoulder, as well as the upper back and triceps (upper-arm) muscles. Strengthening these muscles will help with movements done over your head, such as reaching for or placing objects on high shelves.

Starting position: You may do this exercise standing or seated in a chair. Your back should be straight and your head in line with your spine. Hold the dumbbells with palms facing out, shoulder-width apart or slightly more, at the level of your neck. Your thumbs will be pointing toward your neck. Relax your shoulders down your back.

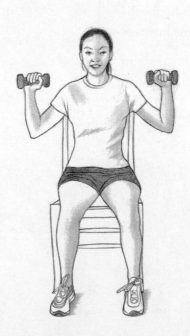

1-2-Up: Press the weights up over your head in a straight line. Do not lock your elbows. Your arms will be above your head and just slightly in front of the plane of your body.

Pause for 1 second, relaxing your shoulders.

1-2-3-Down: Lower the weights to the starting position.

Reps and sets: Repeat the move 12 times—this is 1 set. Rest for about 30 seconds and then do a second set.

Focal points: Keep your upper trunk still during the movement. Initiate the movement in the shoulders. Do not arch your back. The weight is too heavy if you cannot lift it over your head without arching your back. Visualize your shoulders traveling down as you press up. When holding the

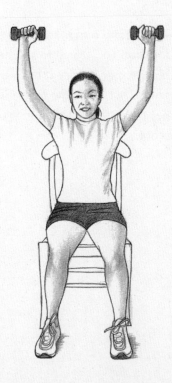

weight, keep your wrist neutral. Avoid letting the weight bring the wrist into extension or flexion.

Progressions

1. Practice the exercise without weight until you can do 12 repetitions in good form. Then start with a 1- to 3-pound weight in each hand and increase the weight by 1 pound per workout until the intensity is a four on the scale after 2 sets of 12 repetitions.

2. As you become stronger and the intensity decreases below a four, increase the weight of the dumbbells by 1- to 3-pound increments per workout to reach a four on the intensity scale.

Modifications: If you have any shoulder or elbow pain, try rotating your palms toward your neck for the starting position, and maintain this position throughout the lift. Also try keeping your hands shoulder-width apart and no further.

Other strength-training modifications and substitutions

Hip abduction and hip adduction (described in the hip osteoarthritis section, pages 124–128) can be alternated every other workout with the knee extension and the knee flexion. This will allow you to incorporate some hip work without losing the knee flexion and extension yet without adding two more exercises to your workout.

Aerobic activity variations

To keep your aerobic program alive and well, you can vary the type of exercise you do. Try a stationary machine if you have been walking, or vice versa. You can also vary the intensity. Do a longer workout (40–60 minutes) once a week at a lower intensity, say, level 2 on the intensity scale. Do a high intensity workout—level 4—for 20 minutes once a week.

Flexibility variations

There is not a lot of room for varying the intensity of a stretch, but you certainly can vary the stretch itself or increase the length of time that you hold it. There are many different stretches for the same muscle group. Look under "Resources" for more stretching ideas.

Yoga, by the way, is a great way to gain flexibility and strength, and you can learn new poses to add to your stretching routine. Classes are widely available. Talk to the instructor to see if the class is appropriate for you. Iyengar yoga can be especially good for those with arthritis because props are used to help support poses for those who are less flexible or have injuries or conditions that limit their range of motion. Chapter 9 has more on yoga, and the "Resources" section has recommendations for yoga videos.

We have learned through our research at Tufts that very specific exercises can reduce arthritis pain and improve overall quality of life for arthritis sufferers. As Liz says, "I used to sleep 9 or 10 hours a night and still wake up tired. But now I can get by on 8 hours a night. I definitely have more energy. And so many things that people take for granted, like being able to pump gas, being able to lie in a field and smell the grass and look up at the sky—I couldn't get myself down on the ground before. Before, a lot of times I'd plan my grocery trips so the boys could be home and help me get stuff into the house. I had to make so many adjustments. Now, it's a pretty normal life."

Triggering Change

■

"I went through enormous periods of ups and downs and a lot of depression," says Liz. "There were some really tough times. I didn't want to get out of bed in the morning. Of course, when you're in a lot of pain, you don't want to use your body. I tried sporadically to do weights at home, but I didn't stick with it. Yet I knew I needed to turn my life around. I wasn't happy with myself."

As you read in Chapter 5, Liz is now very fit and lives a full, active life. She was able to overcome the barriers that were keeping her from changing her habits. But it took a lot of determination and mental work to make it happen. How did she tap into that determination? Most experts only tell you what exercises you should do and which foods to eat. Few provide the critical motivational information you need to start and stick with the program. That is what this chapter is all about.

CHANGE IS HARD

You deserve a lot of credit for resolving to start an exercise program and eat better. That in itself is a big step. But it's important to recognize that adopting any new health behavior requires a pretty big shift in thinking—and doing. Think back to a behavioral change that you made. Perhaps you gave up smoking, decided to floss your teeth every night, or started wearing a seat belt every single time you got in the car. Now think back to what finally made you change. What made the difference?

Like a lot of people, maybe you assume making such a change is all about willpower. You dive into something, and either it works or it doesn't. Then, if you don't stick with it, you've proven to yourself that you're weak-willed and might as well give up before you try again. But willpower's only a small part of change. It takes other things, too, including a plan, whether you're aware of that plan or not.

"It's hard enough to accomplish something even when you have a good plan," says James Prochaska, a University of Rhode Island psychology professor who has specialized in studying how people alter their behavior. "Without a firm plan, forget it."

He likens it to trying to get through the Boston Marathon on sheer willpower. If you haven't planned for the race by gradually increasing the number of miles you run at a time, regularly performing stretches to keep muscles loose and flexible, and eating right and getting enough sleep, "Good luck, willpower," he says.

Now, back to the important change you made in your own life. Chances are that it involved a combination of two things above and beyond willpower: knowledge about how important the behavior change was for your health *and,* consciously or unconsciously, a definitive plan to make it happen, perhaps even a plan that you developed as you went along.

Fortunately, research on changing health behaviors has come a long way in the past several years, and we are going to give you the latest strategies to develop your own plan so that your success will be *guaranteed.*

Accept up front that it takes a little time and effort to set the foundation for long-term success before jumping into the program. It takes asking yourself the right questions. It takes writing lists and keeping logs. Believe us, it's the little steps you first work out on paper that get you there in the long run, taking you out of the psychological mind-set that can make tackling a big change seem so overwhelming.

How ready are you for change?

Change occurs across a continuum. You don't go to bed one night mired in a particular way of life and wake up the next morning ready to do things differently. That's true even for people who stick to their New Year's resolutions. They were preparing long before December 31, whether they realized it or not.

There are actually five phases to the process of change, as outlined by Prochaska. But credit for applying these stages to the development of an exercise program goes to an exceptional behavioral scientist named Bess Marcus from Brown University. Understanding which phase you are in is crucial to determining the best strategies for behavior change.

How ready are you for change?

To find out how ready you are to make significant changes in your lifestyle, select the statement below that best describes you:

1. I am not thinking about changing my eating or activity habits.
2. I am thinking about changing my habits, and I intend to start changing in the next 6 months.
3. I am thinking about changing my habits, and I intend to start changing during the next month.
4. I am already making some changes in my habits (e.g., I lift weights once a week; I eat fish once a week).
5. I have recently changed my behavior, and I am doing what I am supposed to do (e.g., I lift weights three times per week, walk several times per week, and eat plenty of fruits and vegetables).
6. I have successfully changed my behavior, and I have maintained this new behavior for more than 6 months.

If you selected item one, you are in the precontemplation stage. If you selected item two or three, you are in the contemplation stage and may be ready to change. If you selected item four, you are in the preparation stage. If you selected item five, you are in action. If you selected item six, you are in maintenance.

What do these stages really mean?

Precontemplation

Precontemplation is not even realizing that exercise and good nutrition can make a difference in how you live with arthritis. Therefore, you have no motivation to change. The good news is that if you have read any of the earlier chapters in this book, you're definitely past this point and therefore are already *in* the process of change.

Contemplation

This is the stage in which you acquire knowledge that physical activity and nutrition can make a difference in your health, and you begin to think seriously about starting to exercise and eat better. In our experience at Tufts, we find that this is the most difficult stage for people to move out of, because the next stage requires some concerted, organized planning.

Preparation

It's in this stage that you develop a firm, detailed scheme for action. For instance, this is the time that you go to the store and buy the weights. You also sit down with your schedule and plan when you are going to exercise. Perhaps you find a close friend you can count on to join you for walks several times a week. You may have even started initiating some of the changes, like making sure to eat at least 3 servings of vegetables every day or exercising on occasion.

Action

This is the stage at which you actually start to exercise and eat better on a regular basis. You have set a routine, but you have followed it for fewer than 6 months. Therefore, it is not entirely engrained in your lifestyle, like brushing your teeth or putting on your seat belt. The great part about the action stage is that you are starting to feel better. You may have less pain and more energy, which only boost your motivation to continue.

Maintenance

At this stage, the new action becomes second nature, and you will stick with it for the rest of your life. You don't have to remind yourself or force yourself to do it. The reward of the exercise and good nutrition so outweighs any challenges that you wouldn't think of *not* living this way. Of course, life being what it is, you may sometimes have some temporary setbacks when you are sick or your work schedule gets out of hand, but you always return to your routine as soon as you can.

TRIGGERS MAKE CHANGE HAPPEN

There are many barriers that keep us from changing our behaviors—those that we create for ourselves and those that are placed in front of us because of life circumstances. Bess Marcus says that all of these barriers to change start with certain *triggers.* These triggers lead to particular *behaviors,* which engender certain *results.*

Triggers can be positive or negative. Of course, when they set up barriers to better living, they're negative, and they lead to negative results. The goal here is to create positive triggers that lead to positive results. There are five types of triggers.

Cognitive triggers

Cognitive triggers are based on the way we *interpret* our situations. A common negative trigger is, "I don't have time." That leads to a specific behavior, such as not exercising or not shopping for nutritious foods to cook at home. And that, in turn, leads to a negative result: continuing to live with the same amount of arthritis pain. The trick is to work *consciously* at turning the negative cognitive trigger into a positive one so that you'll get positive behaviors and positive results. One way to turn a negative trigger into a positive one might be to say to yourself, "I need time to relax at the end of the day by watching television, but exercise is a greater priority. Two evenings a week I will turn off the television to strength-train—I don't mind missing a couple of sitcoms."

TV and strength training: Great combination or dangerous diversion?

We have said in the past—and still do at times—that strength training can be done while watching television. The rationale behind this recommendation is that many people have trouble finding the right time to strength-train as well as sticking with it once they get started. Combining strength training with a television program you watch regularly, such as the evening news, can create the perfect "habit" many people need to continue with an exercise program long-term.

However, doing strengthening exercises while distracted, as is the case with watching television, *is* less than ideal. With aerobic exercise there is less of a concern because it is a constant, rhythmic motion in which form is generally not much of an issue. But in the case of strength training, you need to be more aware of your body position (form) as well as lifting speed and proper breathing, and that can be a lot to pay attention to, especially when you're just getting started. In addition, watching television while strength training could have consequences such as failing to lift at a high enough intensity, losing track of sets and repetitions, and experiencing a lack of focus that could lead to injuries.

So what's the final word? If you know that the only way you'll strength-train regularly is with the television set on, that is your best option. We recommend that when you're first starting out, limit distractions as best you can and be very attentive to form and speed. Thereafter, try to do at least one or two sessions per week without the television on. During those sessions, count out loud and occasionally check your form in a mirror or with a partner.

Emotional triggers

Depression, guilt, fear, and sadness are all emotions that tend to serve as negative triggers. For instance, if you feel guilty that you're not doing more to help yourself, it gets all too easy to spend your mental energy berating yourself for how little you've accomplished. And then you wind up not embarking on any changes because, "What's the point? I'm so far behind, anyway."

But you can turn the guilt inside out. What if you said to yourself, "I might as well start somewhere. It doesn't feel like taking a small step is going to undo all my sedentary living and poor eating habits, but at least I'll be doing something positive for myself, so I'll feel less guilty." That small step can be anything from having a small baked potato instead of a large order of fries to doing *one* strength-training exercise just once a week. Even if that behavior change doesn't lead to others, you'll end up better off—and maybe in less joint pain—than you would otherwise. It's a very important first step. And just imagine if that one positive change *does* motivate you to try others— which is what we have often found to be the case with our volunteers at Tufts.

Environmental triggers

Where are you going to keep your dumbbells and ankle cuffs? Are you going to store them downstairs when you prefer to exercise upstairs in the bedroom? Even the slight inconvenience of having to take a couple of minutes to run downstairs—or to another room—could be all it takes to trigger a negative set of events, which results in your not exercising and strengthening the muscles that could relieve pressure on your joints.

It's the same with joining a health club. If you join a really snazzy one with all the amenities but it's not on your commuting route, you might never go there after you sign up. You'd be better off joining a fitness club—even without the sauna and Jacuzzi—that doesn't require a detour.

Environmental food triggers can also send you down the path of negative behavior. Maybe you walk to work past a lovely bakery each day, and the delicious aromas waft out and you can't resist a chocolate-filled croissant. If that is the case, you need to find a different route—even if it's more circuitous—to remove this negative trigger. Presto! Instant environmental control that leads to a positive behavior: You get more exercise *and* consume fewer calories.

Physical triggers

A physical trigger like having too much pain in your joints to exercise seems like a reasonable excuse not to pick up your weights or put on your sneakers. But what if, without denying your pain, you reminded yourself that if you exercised, starting out at a low level that does not increase your pain, you would start to feel better and eventually have less pain—as well as other physical benefits. For instance, you would sleep more deeply, which would afford you more energy the next day. Trading in the negative trigger for a positive one removes what for many people is a substantial barrier to physical activity.

Social triggers

Social triggers are the ways in which your behavior is influenced by others. If eating out with a particular person tends to make you anxious and leads to overeating, you might not want to eat out with that person very often. By the same token, if you've chosen an exercise partner who often is unavailable to exercise, you might want to choose a different exercise partner who is as committed as you are—or just do exercises on your own, or enlist a third partner who will motivate both of you.

Family members can have a lot to do with social triggers. Liz's husband was emotionally supportive. However, it was actually her sister-in-law who identified a qualified personal trainer and her father-in-law who paid for some sessions at home until she became comfortable with the idea of going to a gym. That is, Liz had a strong family network that allowed for a constellation of positive social triggers.

You may not have a lot of encouraging family members. But you can make sure to surround yourself with supportive (or at least not sabotaging) friends, as well as health-care providers. For instance, if your doctor believes only in pills and discourages you from strength training or better eating because he or she says they won't help you, you may want to find a doctor who is enthusiastic and encouraging about the behaviors you want to try.

WRITE IT DOWN

We have found that the best way to identify your negative triggers is to keep a simple diary: nothing fancy—more like a log, really. You may not want to spend this time before you get started, but it will actually *save* time by helping you bypass setbacks once you've begun. That's because it will point out things about your life that are likely to trip you up, so you can be prepared with solutions in advance. The diary will lead you out of the contemplation stage and well into the preparation stage—the stage just before "action," or as action is beginning. We ask that you fill it out for 2 weekdays and 1 weekend day to get an idea of your habits. If you want to fill it out for more days, please do.

The diary should have three components:

1. *Keep track of your activities, physical as well as sedentary.* What did you do during your lunch hour, for instance? Did you do any gardening? Did you walk the dog at night or just let the pooch into the yard? Did you strength-train or participate in any sports activities? Aside from writing down the activity, include the factors that surrounded the activity, such as time, location, weather, people you were with, whether it was a workday or not, etc.

2. *Record your food habits.* Remember, it doesn't have to be elaborate. Just write down all the food you ate during the day. Make sure that you record whether it was a meal that you sat down to or just a snack. Also include whether or not you ate with others, what time of day the meals or snacks were consumed, and whether you were at home, at work, or somewhere else.

3. *Write down your feelings.* As we've said above, your emotions as well as how you process your thoughts have a lot to do with the behaviors you engage in. You'll learn whether "I feel fat" makes you eat more or less, whether "I don't have time" stops you from rearranging activities to *create* more time, and whether positive thoughts such as "I feel strong today" help you to be more active.

Taking these three steps will help you discern a pattern—or lack thereof—in how you manage your time, and they'll also get you thinking about what triggers your various activities.

Activity, Food, and Feelings Diary

WEEKDAY 1

Activity patterns (includes sedentary and leisure activities as well as planned exercise):

_____

_____

_____

_____

Eating habits:

_____

_____

_____

_____

Feelings (both positive and negative):

_____

_____

_____

_____

WEEKDAY 2

Activity patterns (includes sedentary and leisure activities as well as planned exercise):

_____

_____

_____

_____

Eating habits:

_____
_____
_____

Feelings (both positive and negative):

_____
_____
_____
_____

WEEKEND DAY

Activity patterns (includes sedentary and leisure activities as well as planned exercise):

_____
_____
_____

Eating habits:

_____
_____
_____
_____

Feelings (both positive and negative):

_____
_____
_____

Identifying your triggers

Once you have spent several days on this task, you will be ready to identify *in writing* your five types of triggers—cognitive, emotional, environmental, physical, and social—for the behaviors in which you engage. Look at times you exercised and ate well. Try to identify the factors, or triggers, that are associated with those positive behaviors. Now, look at the times you didn't exercise or eat well. Again, try to figure out the triggers.

Let's say, for example, that you buy fast food for lunch three times a week. Perhaps it will become clear to you that the trigger is an environmental one—the variety of fast-food places near your place of work. Or maybe it's cognitive: "I don't have time to bring a sandwich from home" or "Healthy food is too expensive." Or social: "My friends always eat at the same place."

Putting your finger on the negative trigger makes it easier to shift to a positive one: "There are more healthful restaurants nearby, and even though the food costs more, the extra ten or twenty dollars a week is worth it if it helps me to eat better." *Or,* "It takes about 20 minutes for me to run out and come back with a burger. It would take me less time to prepare a tuna sandwich at home or bring in wholesome leftovers." *Or,* "I enjoy lunchtime with my friends, so maybe I can convince them to eat the way *I* want to once or twice a week *or* take a walk with me instead of going over to the drive-through *or* just have lunch on my own sometimes even though I will miss the socializing."

If eating on your own is something you just can't do, and if convincing your friends to spend lunchtime differently is something you just can't make happen, think about how you might be able to turn "cannots" into "cans." Perhaps the solution is to go with your friends to the burger place but to bring a fruit from home and have that instead of fries. It's a trade-off, but maybe one you could live with more easily.

Whatever you decide to do, these solutions are all about exchanging certain triggers and behaviors for ones that will better help you reach your larger goal—to feel better both physically and emotionally. It's not always a snap. There's a difference between "wanting" something and "being prepared to pay a price for it." But by working through these trade-offs before you start, you actually *increase* your resolve, or willpower, because you strengthen your commitment to the change.

The top-ten negative triggers . . . and how to solve them

Here are the ten most common negative triggers we have heard from the people we have worked with at Tufts . . . and the positive triggers they substituted to help develop new behaviors—and health-enhancing outcomes.

I don't have time (cognitive)

Eating right and exercising regularly have to become a priority in your schedule. Take a look at the diary you just filled out—or at your calendar. Find at least two times during the week when you know you can make room to fit in a workout. Write down the times on your calendar. Make it a priority, like an important business meeting. If there is a time when your children watch a specific television show a couple of times a week, make that your trigger to go exercise.

I am too tired (physical)

The reality here is that you probably *are* tired. But if you start exercising and eating better, you are going to have much more energy *and* you are going to sleep better. Choose a time to exercise when you are least tired.

I am too unhealthy to exercise (physical)

It is true that if you have an unstable medical condition, you shouldn't start to exercise until you have worked closely with your doctor to get the problem under control. But most people can start our program even if they have multiple medical conditions or are overweight or elderly. At Tufts we have worked with hundreds of people with various chronic diseases and have found without exception that exercise and eating right help to reduce the signs and symptoms of disease—and make you healthier.

My friends and family are not supportive (social)

You need to find those friends and family members who do understand your needs and can take an active interest in helping you. No one can take responsibility for your change in behaviors except you. But friends and family can give you the needed support to make the change happen. You may even hire a personal trainer to assist you a couple of times a week to help you out. Miriam has her best friends come over on Saturday mornings to lift weights with her. "I know I will always lift weights at least that one day," she says, "and I really enjoy catching up on the weekly events."

I get bored exercising (cognitive)

There are several ways to enhance your exercise routine. Choose activities that suit your interests. Exercise to music that you really enjoy. Change your routine around as we have outlined in the exercise program. Take an exercise class that introduces you to new people and new moves.

I don't have enough money to exercise or eat well (environmental)

It doesn't cost as much as you think; you don't have to join a fancy gym or buy gourmet food. You can purchase second-hand weights through the classified ads or share them with a friend. And you can buy fruits and vegetables in season or eat some frozen and canned foods. Remember, too, that it costs a lot more to be sick and dependent on others than to buy the foods and exercise equipment that will improve your health.

Healthful food doesn't taste good (cognitive)

Many people think that healthful food must taste bad. That isn't true. No matter what your tastes are, you can find healthful dishes that taste good to you.

Eating right and adding exercise just piles more stress onto my busy life (emotional)

Exercise is perhaps the best stress *reliever*. Research study after research study has shown that when people start exercising, their stress levels are diminished and their coping mechanisms enhanced.

I don't have anywhere to go to exercise (environmental)

One of the benefits of our exercise program is that you can strength-train at home. And if you don't have easily available safe roads or sidewalks for the aerobic component of the exercise program, you can probably find a mall, high school track, or a walking trail near your home. Alternatively, you can purchase a stationary treadmill or cycle. Look for used ones in your newspaper's classified section. We find, however, that going outside for your aerobic workouts is very satisfying and relaxing. So, whenever possible, try to get outside and enjoy your surroundings.

I don't like to cook (physical)

There are healthful convenience foods available today that make eating better on the go easier: prepackaged salads, whole-grain breads, even delicious entrées like burritos with beans at "natural foods" stores and many supermarkets. Find a local natural foods store that carries more healthful alternatives to some of your usual quick fare, and browse the prepared-foods section. Frozen vegetables are a great substitute for fresh when washing, cutting, and cooking seem too daunting.

SETTING GOALS THAT MOTIVATE YOU EVEN MORE

Setting goals is crucial. They will help you put the icing on the preparation cake, so to speak. You can't just say, "I'm going to exercise more" or "I'm going to eat better" once you've come up with positive triggers to help you live more healthfully. Shifts in lifestyle require an organizing principle based on goals that are very specific—as well as reasonable. If you've never exercised in your life, a goal to start strength training for 40 minutes three times a week and engaging in 20 minutes of aerobic activities another three times a week is not going to serve you. The difference between "here" and "there" is just too great, and you'll give up because of the overwhelming task you've set for yourself. A better short-term goal: "I will walk for 5 minutes after dinner three nights a week for 4 weeks. I will do 15 minutes of strength training three times a week." That's plenty right there (and exactly what we recommend) for someone who has been sedentary for decades. It's also specific enough that you can keep track on paper whether you're accomplishing what you set out to do.

Similarly, for dietary goals, be realistic. If you never eat fish right now and fewer than six fruits and vegetables per day, your goal should be to eat fish twice over the next 3 weeks and increase your produce intake by 1 serving a day—or even 1 serving every few days.

Once the 3 weeks have passed, you can evaluate how you feel about what you've been doing. Do you need to drop back a bit? Does it feel like the right amount? Are you ready to add more walking time or more strength-training sessions?

You can always reevaluate your goals as you go, but the more you can break them down into small steps, the less overwhelming they will seem. In addition, the better you'll be able to chart your progress (keeping a log of your exercise and eating habits, particularly at first, is a great motivator as you keep checking things off), and the more your new habits will become integrated into your daily life without much thought. Then, too, if you see that you did something eight times and missed it only twice, you'll be able to "get right back on the horse" rather than feel you've "blown it," because you'll see that a lapse here and there doesn't ruin a routine.

Finally, and this is very important, make sure you set for yourself "I will do" goals rather than "I will be" goals. You can't will yourself to *be* a certain weight or *at* a particular level of fitness. But you can set goals for how much exercise you will do and how often—as well as for what you will eat and when. Those are things over which you have full control. And they'll edge you toward your broader goals without anxiety because you'll be accomplishing something every single time you stick to your plan. You don't have to let everything ride on one weigh-in or one "final" fitness session.

THE REWARDS OF YOUR EFFORTS

For some people, the rewards are the positive results that come from the new positive behaviors—feeling better, looking better, having a sense of accomplishment. Says Sister Mary Patrice about her strength-training regimen, "The improvement in my walk, the improvement in pain, was so different. I felt so much better."

These are *internal* rewards, and they will no doubt be your greatest ones. Some people, however, when they reach goals that they set for themselves, like to give themselves *external* rewards, too. We think that's great. Why shouldn't you treat yourself a little special for hard-won accomplishments? Such rewards can even help spur you on to new goals.

That's why, for example, if shoes are your thing, you're entitled to a new pair for a particular goal that you've reached. Perhaps you walked every night after dinner for 3 weeks. Or maybe you'd prefer tickets to a sports event or a weekend away with your spouse or friend. Whatever your "gold star" for success in your efforts, you deserve it.

———

We know you can do it—and that the rewards will come. We have seen people who have never exercised in their entire lives start with small steps and then get very strong over time. They also begin to try new foods that they never thought they would eat and actually wind up enjoying the taste and the added health benefits. Remember that the steps are small at first. That's how Liz handled it—step by step. She started out doing leg lifts with only about 3 pounds on each leg. "It was hard," she says, "because my range of motion was really limited." It didn't feel to her like she was doing anything for herself. But those small steps have led to a much more pain-free life filled not just with mundane chores but also with activities that she loves, including climbing mountains and bicycling through the countryside.

Supportive Therapies

CHAPTER 7

Choosing the Right Medication(s)

■

A lot of people don't like to take pills. They feel that relying on a drug to lessen pain or control a condition means they're officially "sick," that they've engaged in a battle of wills with an illness and that the illness has won out and proven just how sick they are.

Nothing could be further from the truth. What if you're doing everything you can with both exercise and nutrition to control your arthritis, and engaging in the positive thinking that we described in the previous chapter, yet still cannot control your pain or the progression of your disease? Then talking with your doctor about taking a medication to complement the lifestyle changes you've made is a sign of *strength*. It means you're doing everything in your power to strong-arm your body into letting you live as full a life as possible. It means you're taking advantage of a very powerful option at your disposal. We feel strongly that sound medication management is a critical component when it comes to maximizing your results with our exercise and nutrition program.

Fortunately, there are literally dozens of medications to help control the course of the disease, or at least lessen the pain, and better ones are hitting the market all the time. That's particularly good news in light of the fact that not all drugs are equally effective—or appropriate—for all people. Some people may be more vulnerable than others to the side effects of one or another drug. Then, too, there are cost considerations. Some medications are much more expensive than others, and in many cases a less expensive one will work just as well.

If you're working with a good physician, he or she will tell you all about a drug, what it will do (as well as won't do), possible side effects, and how long you should try it to see if it helps before switching to another (you don't take it forever if it's not working). But the more you know about the arthritis drugs that are out there to begin with, the better equipped you'll be to act as a *partner* in health-care decisions concerning whether to take a particular medication(s).

In this chapter, we outline virtually all the drugs available for the treatment of arthritis. You'll learn what they do, what they don't do, *how* they do it, their side effects (and how to counteract them), cost considerations, and other salient points.

DRUGS THAT CONTROL PAIN

For both osteoarthritis and rheumatoid arthritis as well as other inflammatory forms of the disease, including lupus and ankylosing spondylitis, two large classes of medications control painful symptoms: nonsteroidal anti-inflammatory drugs (NSAIDs) and steroids.

Nonsteroidal anti-inflammatory drugs (NSAIDs)

There are about twenty-five different NSAIDs available. And while none of them stems erosion of the joints, what they do accomplish—relief from pain and some reduction in swelling and stiffness—is no small thing.

NSAIDs work by reducing inflammation at the joint site. Inflammation can cause pain in a couple of different ways. For instance, the white blood cells that contribute to inflammation may irritate sensitive nerve endings. In addition, the white cells cause fluid buildup, which is part and parcel of inflammation and stretches the joint capsule (tissue that surrounds the entire joint). That stretching, in turn, "activates" pain receptors. NSAIDs blunt inflammation to some degree by blocking production of prostaglandins—those small molecules produced by white blood cells that stimulate inflammatory activity.

Some of the pain relief comes fast—you'll get your pain down from a "10" to an "8" pretty much during the first few days that you take the drug (see Workbook page 252 for the pain scale). That's because NSAIDs provide some direct analgesic, or pain-relieving, effect. But the pain won't go down to, say, a "2" until the actual anti-inflammatory effect kicks in. And that takes 2–4 weeks because you need to build up a therapeutic amount of the drug in your joints.

Thus, even if you don't get dramatic relief from an NSAID in the first 10–14 days, don't give up on it. And don't skip doses! *You have to take an NSAID regularly, not just when you're in pain.* Those people who take NSAIDS in sporadic fashion lose out on most of their benefit. NSAIDs are transferred from the bloodstream to the joints via "diffusion," meaning that they go naturally from an area of high NSAID concentration to an area of low concentration. If you miss a dose, the concentration in the bloodstream drops, so the NSAID that has built up in the joints travels back out to the blood. From there, it goes to the kidneys and is excreted in the urine.

Because it's necessary to take NSAIDs regularly to get their full benefit, you might want to select a longer-acting drug that can be taken once or twice a day rather than three or four times—it'll be easier to stick to the regimen. However, the longer-acting drugs are often more expensive. It's a trade-off you need to keep in mind as you choose.

NSAIDs and the risk of gastrointestinal bleeding

While NSAIDs are remarkable in their ability to reduce inflammation and, thereby, pain, they come with a significant potential hazard when taken on a regular basis: internal bleeding in the gastrointestinal tract. Such bleeding may produce no obvious symptoms at first, but it could be draining your body of vital blood cells. Aspirin, the original NSAID (and just as effective at reducing inflammation as any other), is particularly hard on the stomach. Bleeding from chronic long-term use of aspirin, as well as from other NSAIDs, can take the form of gastritis or an ulcer.

The reason that NSAIDs can cause bleeding, ulcers, or gastritis in the stomach and intestine turns out to be the same reason that they can help your joints. It's all in their ability to reduce prostaglandins. While prostaglandins contribute to inflammation, they are also crucial for making the stomach wall acid-proof. Specifically, prostaglandins send important signals to the stomach to make a mucous lining that prevents acid from attacking, and in

Cox-2 inhibitors for people at high risk for bleeding

Those at high risk for bleeding will probably be told by their doctors that they should take rofecoxib (Vioxx) or celecoxib (Celebrex). These two drugs are the first of a new generation of NSAIDs, called *Cox-2 inhibitors,* that present a much lower risk for bleeding than other NSAIDs. How are they different? They reduce only the "bad" prostaglandins that contribute to inflammation and leave the "good" stomach-protecting prostaglandins alone.

Prostaglandins are activated by a type of enzyme known as *cyclo-oxygenase,* or "Cox" for short. There are two types of Cox enzymes: Cox-1 stimulates the prostagladins that send signals to coat the stomach lining with protective mucus and perform various other beneficial functions in the body; Cox-2 stimulates the inflammation-causing prostaglandins in white blood cells.

Most NSAIDs inhibit all prostaglandins, the "good" and the "bad." But Cox-2 inhibitors, as their name suggests, inhibit only the bad, inflammatory ones, so people who take them have reduced inflammation—and pain—in their joints yet do not suffer from stomach bleeding.

The drawback is that Cox-2 inhibitors are much more expensive than other NSAIDs—five to ten times more expensive. They cost about three dollars a day, or more than $1,000 a year, and many insurance plans do not cover them unless less expensive NSAIDs have been tried and didn't work, or have proven to be a problem, *or* your doctor can demonstrate that you have a high risk for bleeding.

Age increases the risk of gastrointestinal bleeding (as well as other NSAID side effects), but age alone doesn't make a case for needing a Cox-2 inhibitor. Most U.S. insurance plans currently demand that you have a history of ulcers or other evidence of gastrointestinal bleeding—or evidence of being prone to it.

Fortunately, even if you are not a candidate for one of the Cox-2 inhibitors yet show signs of stomach trouble upon taking one of the other NSAIDs, there are drugs that can counter that effect while allowing NSAIDs to do their work of reducing inflammation in joints. See the information on page 197 for details.

Note: Recent evidence suggests that Cox-2 inhibitors do not protect people from heart disease the way old-fashioned aspirin does. They potentially could even *increase* the risk for heart disease in some people, as reported in the August 2001 issue of the *Journal of the American Medical Association.* As this book goes to press, there is not enough evidence to know whether or not this is a serious problem. It has to be balanced against the much higher risk for intestinal bleeding in people with a history of ulcers or gastritis. Our advice is to discuss this with your doctor and take mini-dose aspirin along with your Cox-2 inhibitor if he or she suggests it. "Baby aspirin" (81 milligrams per day) will protect most people against heart disease without harming the stomach.

some cases eating away at, the stomach wall. Without that prostaglandin signal, the stomach becomes very vulnerable.

Gastritis, the most common side effect of reduced prostaglandins, consists of redness and swelling of the stomach lining. But ulcers occur with some frequency, too. *Ulcer* is the medical term for a hole (in this case burned through tissue by acid), and it can occur either in the stomach (*gastric ulcer*) or the duodenum, which is the upper part of the small intestine (*duodenal ulcer*). Both gastric and duodenal ulcers are known as *peptic ulcers.*

Whatever the condition that may accompany the bleeding, the speed at which you bleed determines the severity of the situation. If you bleed quickly, which is rare, you could be in a life-threatening situation of losing too much blood. Much more common is a slow bleed that leads to problems such as anemia, which causes weakness and fatigue.

Some people are at a much higher risk than others for internal bleeding from NSAIDs. For instance, somebody with a history of peptic ulcers is more likely to bleed taking NSAIDs than someone without such a history.

Other NSAID side effects

While gastrointestinal bleeding is the most common side effect of taking NSAIDs, it's not the only possible one. There are some other common adverse reactions, and they can occur with Cox-2 inhibitors as well as with all the other NSAIDs.

- *Hypersensitivity/allergic response:* People who have asthma or nasal polyps tend to be allergic to aspirin and sometimes to other NSAIDs, too. In fact, sometimes they are instructed to take their first dose right in the doctor's office so that they can be injected with a needle of epinephrine should the NSAID close up their breathing passages.
- *Increased propensity to bleed:* NSAIDs lengthen the time it takes for blood to clot, which could present a serious problem in the case of an accident or emergency surgery. Aspirin is the most potent inhibitor of blood clotting, although the other NSAIDs lengthen blood-clotting time as well. Still, it is not a common enough problem to make people in pain avoid NSAIDs.
- *Liver "irritation":* Liver function can become compromised, so periodic blood tests that measure liver function should be conducted. Again, stopping the drug generally reverses the damage.
- *Rash:* Every drug ever made has caused a rash in somebody. The rashes are generally itchy red spots on the legs and trunk that go away when the medicine is stopped. Not all NSAIDs cause rashes in the same person, but if one causes a rash on you, you may have to try other NSAIDs until your doctor finds one that doesn't give you skin problems.
- *Reduced kidney function:* Fortunately, out-and-out kidney failure is rare. Moreover, it often takes years for much damage to occur, and stopping the drug usually reverses the damage. But some people have an immediate reaction to NSAIDs in their kidneys, so we recommend having a blood test to check kidney function about 2–4 weeks after starting these medicines.

We should note that some arthritis experts argue that NSAIDs actually accelerate the pace of the disease because the relief from pain that they achieve makes people too hard on their eroding joint(s). But we feel that at best it's a controversial opinion. Let's say you need a hip joint replaced

6 months earlier than otherwise if you take NSAIDs. The upside is that you will have had up to 5 years more function from the original hip joint. It's a trade-off worth making.

Drugs to prevent G.I. bleeding from NSAIDs

NSAIDs cause gastrointestinal bleeding and other stomach problems such as ulcers because they stop the buildup of the mucous lining that protects the stomach wall from acid secreted there to help digest food. But is it possible to continue taking NSAIDs to reduce joint pain even if they're making the stomach much less able to withstand the acid onslaught and therefore more likely to bleed? Yes, if you really need them. The antidote is to take medications that can protect the stomach lining. The most common medications to prevent gastrointestinal bleeding from NSAIDs are those that reduce acid in the stomach. These medications include ranitidine (Zantac), cimetidine (Tagamet), nizatidine (Axid), famotidine (Pepcid), omeprazol (Prilosec), lensoprazole (Prevacid), misoprostol (Cytotec), and sucralfate (Carafate).

Granted, it is not ideal to prescribe a second drug to treat the side effects of the first, but often there is no choice. Even the new Cox-2 inhibitors can cause stomach upset, even if the risk of bleeding is almost zero.

Note that people with diabetes seem to be at relatively high risk for NSAID-induced bleeding and ulcers; they appear to have trouble with blood flow to the stomach. If you have diabetes and are taking NSAIDs, you should discuss with your doctor whether to take a drug that reduces stomach acid.

Nineteen common NSAIDs

Listed below are nineteen of the most commonly taken NSAIDs. Included are their brand names, generic names, the best type of candidate for each drug, cost per 30 days, how hard each drug is on the stomach, and notes, when appropriate, that include particular side effects or what to ask your doctor. Be aware as well that the prescribed doses can very considerably from one person to the next, depending on such factors as age, body size, and disease severity.

All NSAIDs, we want to note, can worsen existing kidney or liver problems or heart failure. And pregnant women should not take NSAIDs in the third trimester or during breast feeding—they cross over to the milk to some extent. Women should also not take these drugs earlier in pregnancy unless they have the approval of a physician.

Note, too, that NSAIDs can interact with many other medications, either increasing or decreasing their potency, so make sure your doctor knows all the medicines you are taking before you start on a new one, including herbal remedies and over-the-counter drugs.

Interestingly, some of the drugs listed here are the over-the-counter version of prescription drugs listed in the same chart. For instance, Aleve is the over-the-counter version of naproxen. What makes one drug a prescription medicine and another an over-the-counter preparation? The dosage. Aleve contains 220 milligrams per pill, while naproxen contains 375 or 500 milligrams, which means that you have to take fewer pills a day.

You might think over-the-counter drugs are cheaper than prescription medicines and thus are worth the extra pill popping. But that's not necessarily the case. If you have a health insurance policy that requires only a small copayment for prescription drugs, the prescription version of a drug may very well be cheaper. Granted, the $10–$15 you spend on the copay may equal the price of an over-the-counter bottle, but you go through the over-the-counter bottle faster because you have to take more pills to get the same dose.

Do a little homework before you decide that one version of a drug is a better buy than the other. After comparison shopping, you can rest assured that you are buying the least expensive version of the drug you're supposed to be taking.

$ means the drug costs less than $25 per 30 days (we don't assume you have insurance here—your cost may be much less).

$$ means $25–$49 per 30 days.

$$$ means $50–$99 per 30 days.

$$$$ means $100–$199 per 30 days.

$$$$$ means more than $200 per 30 days.

For "How tough on the stomach," "1" is the least tough; "3," the toughest.

BRAND NAME: Anaprox
GENERIC NAME: naproxen sodium
BEST CANDIDATE: general use
COST PER 30 DAYS: $$$
HOW TOUGH ON THE STOMACH: 2

BRAND NAME: Ansaid
GENERIC NAME: flurbiprofen
BEST CANDIDATE: general use
COST PER 30 DAYS: $$$
HOW TOUGH ON THE STOMACH: 3

BRAND NAME: Celebrex
GENERIC NAME: celecoxib
BEST CANDIDATE: high risk of gastrointestinal bleeding
COST PER 30 DAYS: $$$$
HOW TOUGH ON THE STOMACH: 1
NOTE: Cox-2 inhibitor

BRAND NAME: Clinoril
GENERIC NAME: sulindac
BEST CANDIDATE: may be safer for those whose kidney function is reduced
COST PER 30 DAYS: $$$
HOW TOUGH ON THE STOMACH: 2

BRAND NAME: Daypro
GENERIC NAME: oxaprozin
BEST CANDIDATE: general use
COST PER 30 DAYS: $$$
HOW TOUGH ON THE STOMACH: 2

BRAND NAME: Disalcid
GENERIC NAME: salsalate
BEST CANDIDATE: elderly; people with blood-clotting or bleeding problems
COST PER 30 DAYS: $$
HOW TOUGH ON THE STOMACH: 1

BRAND NAME: Dolobid
GENERIC NAME: diflunisal
BEST CANDIDATE: general use; elderly
COST PER 30 DAYS: $$$
HOW TOUGH ON THE STOMACH: 2

BRAND NAME: Ecotrin, Bayer, and others
GENERIC NAME: aspirin (enteric-coated)
BEST CANDIDATE: younger people
COST PER 30 DAYS: $
HOW TOUGH ON THE STOMACH: 3

BRAND NAME: Feldene
GENERIC NAME: piroxicam
BEST CANDIDATE: younger people
COST PER 30 DAYS: $$$
HOW TOUGH ON THE STOMACH: 2

BRAND NAME: Indocin
GENERIC NAME: indomethacin
BEST CANDIDATE: severe arthritis, gout, spondyloarthritis
COST PER 30 DAYS: $
HOW TOUGH ON THE STOMACH: 3

BRAND NAME: Lodine
GENERIC NAME: etodolac
BEST CANDIDATE: general use
COST PER 30 DAYS: $$$
HOW TOUGH ON THE STOMACH: 2

BRAND NAME: Mobic
GENERIC NAME: meloxicam
BEST CANDIDATE: general use
COST PER 30 DAYS: $$$
HOW TOUGH ON THE STOMACH: 1

BRAND NAME: Motrin, Advil, and others
GENERIC NAME: ibuprofen
BEST CANDIDATE: general use
COST PER 30 DAYS: $
HOW TOUGH ON THE STOMACH: 1

BRAND NAME: Naprosyn, Aleve

GENERIC NAME: naproxen

BEST CANDIDATE: general use

COST PER 30 DAYS: $$$

HOW TOUGH ON THE STOMACH: 2

BRAND NAME: Orudis

GENERIC NAME: ketoprofen

BEST CANDIDATE: general use

COST PER 30 DAYS: $$$

HOW TOUGH ON THE STOMACH: 2

BRAND NAME: Relafen

GENERIC NAME: nabumetone

BEST CANDIDATE: general use; elderly

COST PER 30 DAYS: $$$

HOW TOUGH ON THE STOMACH: 1

BRAND NAME: Trilisate

GENERIC NAME: choline magnesium trisalicylate

BEST CANDIDATE: elderly; people with blood-clotting or bleeding problems

COST PER 30 DAYS: $$$

HOW TOUGH ON THE STOMACH: 1

NOTE: may be used with Coumadin (warfarin) as long as monitored closely

BRAND NAME: Vioxx

GENERIC NAME: rofecoxib

BEST CANDIDATE: history of ulcers or gastrointestinal bleeding

COST PER 30 DAYS: $$$$

HOW TOUGH ON THE STOMACH: 1

NOTE: Cox-2 inhibitor

BRAND NAME: Voltaren

GENERIC NAME: diclofenac sodium

BEST CANDIDATE: general use

COST PER 30 DAYS: $$$

HOW TOUGH ON THE STOMACH: 2

NOTES: Voltaren is also available by the brand name Arthrotec. Arthrotec is a combination of Voltaren and the stomach protector misoprostol (Cytotec), developed for people with gastritis or ulcers and arthritis. It is effective, but often people can get equal stomach protection from an NSAID plus an H2-blocker such as ranitidine (Zantac) or famotidine (Pepcid). There is a convenience in having both drugs in a single pill, but you may have to pay extra for it.

When acetaminophen (Tylenol) should be used instead of an NSAID

Sometimes the pain of arthritis is not due to inflammation, or swelling, at the joint but to the fact that so much cartilage has worn away that bone is scraping on top of bone. In such cases, an NSAID or other anti-inflammatory drug isn't going to be of much use. In fact, you're probably going to need surgery at some point to replace the eroded joint. In the meantime, however, acetaminophen (Tylenol) can help control the pain. (Believe it or not, no one knows how Tylenol works!)

How do you know if your pain is due to inflammation or to total erosion of the joint cartilage? You don't, at least not without your physician's help. A physical examination can identify whether there's excess joint fluid—a sign of inflammation—and an X-ray can tell you how much cartilage has been lost. Once you know the cause of the pain, you know the appropriate medicine.

Do take acetaminophen if your doctor recommends it. It is often used with NSAIDs for extra pain relief. While high doses can cause liver and kidney damage over the long term, those risks are low, particularly for people who will stop taking the drug once they get better—either after surgery or as a result of our program!

Steroids

Like NSAIDs, steroids suppress inflammation, thereby reducing pain and stiffness, but they're more effective. Whereas NSAIDs just stand in the way of a single enzyme to block the production of the prostaglandins involved in inflammation caused by the white blood cells of the immune system, steroids shut down the entire immune system on several biochemical fronts. That's extremely important, since the immune system on overdrive is what causes so many of the problems of arthritic, particularly rheumatoid arthritis and other inflammatory arthritic conditions.

The body actually produces steroids, a type of stress hormone, naturally. One steroid, *cortisol,* works to close down the immune system after it responds to infections so that it doesn't keep running after it has done its job. But people with rheumatoid arthritis, in particular, make less cortisol than others in response to stress, so there's less of a signal to the immune system to shut off. It's as if it's always running "at a simmer."

Enter steroid *drugs,* synthetic steroids that mimic cortisol and thus are very effective at suppressing the pain and stiffness resulting from inflammation. The original synthetic version of cortisol is *cortisone,* which was first manufactured in the 1940s. Since then, a number of other synthetic steroids have been developed, the most well known of which is *prednisone.* They can be taken by mouth, injected directly into the muscles (intramuscular injection) or the bloodstream (intravenous injection), or injected through the skin directly into an afflicted joint (intra-articular injection).

Steroids taken by mouth

Steroids taken by mouth are not prescribed for people who have osteoarthritis. Such steroids are "systemic," meaning they reach the whole body, and, as you'll recall from Chapter 2, osteoarthritis is not a systemic disease.

It tends to target only one or two joints. That's why steroid pills are essentially only for people who have rheumatoid arthritis or lupus or some other type of inflammatory arthritis—conditions in which the entire body can be affected.

Those with rheumatoid arthritis tend to be especially responsive to steroid pills, even in low doses. Sometimes as little as 2–3 milligrams a day is enough to significantly suppress pain and stiffness. With lupus, however, you may need anywhere from 10–100 milligrams daily.

Steroids injected into the muscles or bloodstream

Intramuscular injections are generally used for people with the arthritic condition gout. Attacks of gout, which are caused by a buildup of uric acid inside the joints, tend to occur sporadically, but when they do, they can be very painful. Injections of steroid drugs into the muscles break off an attack of gout within 24–48 hours.

Intravenous steroids are used in life-threatening situations to get a high dose of medicine into someone when the need is critical. Such a need most often arises with lupus and other autoimmune diseases but occasionally with rheumatoid arthritis, too.

Steroids injected directly into an afflicted joint

This kind of injection can be useful for people with rheumatoid arthritis *or* osteoarthritis. It delivers a huge dose of steroids right to the problem and thereby suppresses joint inflammation—and concomitant pain—for anywhere from a few weeks to a few months. It works best the first time, and then not as well thereafter—one of the reasons it's sometimes used before joint replacement surgery. It buys some major pain relief before the operation. It can also buy time if you have switched arthritis medications and have to wait a while for the new drug to kick in.

Steroid side effects

While steroids provide greater pain relief than NSAIDs, they can also cause a longer, and often more serious, list of side effects. Such effects are rare in people who get an injection of steroids directly into a joint because these shots tend to be given only once. Not enough of the drug builds up in the body to cause problems. Much the same is true of injections into muscle. It's steroid *pills,* sometimes taken over the long term (years and even decades), that tend to cause problems, with risks rising with the duration of the pill-taking and the dose of medication. Here are the most common potential side effects:

- *Avascular necrosis of bone:* A potentially catastrophic complication of taking steroids, it means the death of the ends of bone. It occurs most commonly in the hip but can also take place in the knees, ankles, shoulders, or wrists. Once it sets in, joint replacement surgery is usually needed. Fortunately, this complication occurs in only 1–2 percent of patients taking steroids.
- *Cataracts:* You have to be taking steroids for several years before you need to worry that they are going to lead to a cataract. The older the person, the higher the risk.
- *Diabetes:* Steroids cause insulin resistance, which means the body becomes much more resistant to the efforts of the hormone insulin to transfer sugar from the bloodstream to all of the tissues. High sugar levels in the blood are the hallmark of diabetes.
- *Gastric ulcers:* These are uncommon, occurring with much less frequency than they do in people taking NSAIDs, but they are a concern, especially in the elderly. People taking both NSAIDs and steroids are at higher risk, however.
- *Hair thinning:* This occurs on the head.
- *High "bad" LDL-cholesterol, low "good" HDL-cholesterol, and high triglycerides:* All of these contribute to the development of heart disease.
- *Hirsutism:* Hair growth on the face is possible.
- *Infections:* Because steroids are immune suppressants, infections are more likely to take hold. This is particularly true of people taking more than 40 milligrams a day.
- *Oral thrush:* This is a buildup of a fungus, *Candida albicans,* in the mouth, and generally occurs in people who take more than 20 milligrams daily.
- *Obesity:* Steroids promote the storage of fat and the wasting of muscle. They can also cause a craving for sweets, which tend to be high in calories.
- *Osteoporosis:* Even a dose of prednisone as low as 5–10 milligrams

Protecting against steroid-induced osteoporosis

While steroid drugs can decrease bone mass by as much as 10 percent in the first 6 months of therapy, there are clear guidelines for protecting against that possibility. They include taking supplemental doses of calcium and vitamin D, getting periodic bone density scans (particularly important for women and older men), and potentially taking a bone-saving drug such as Fosamax, Evista, Actonel, Miacalcin, or, in the case of older women, hormone replacement therapy (HRT).

Unfortunately, too few medical practitioners are following these guidelines, as researchers at the Medical College of Virginia found when they surveyed 147 patients taking steroids every day for an average of 1–2 years. Only 29 percent of the patients interviewed had had a bone density scan; only 29 percent received calcium supplements; and fewer than half of them took vitamin D.

It takes years of treatment to build up depleted bone mass, which is why working to *prevent* bone loss is so crucial. Here are protective measures you should discuss with your doctor:

- 1,000 milligrams daily of supplemental calcium
- 800 IU daily of vitamin D
- annual bone density scans (DXA scan)
- possible bone-protecting drug treatment
- strength-training exercises
- weight-bearing aerobic exercises

For more information on how to prevent or treat osteoporosis, please see the book *Strong Women, Strong Bones,* written by Miriam Nelson with Sarah Wernick (see "Resources" for a complete citation).

causes calcium losses in the urine, which can lead to long-term thinning of the bones. The lower your bone density when you *start* taking steroids, the greater the chance for steroids to contribute to osteoporosis development. (See the box on page 206 for measures to stave off osteoporosis during steroid treatment.)

- *Psychosis:* Even with high doses (above 40 milligrams a day), steroid-induced psychosis is uncommon. It tends to occur in people who are already prone to mental illness. But taking steroids can lead to vivid dreams or mood swings.
- *Striae:* These are similar to stretch marks on the belly or thighs.

DRUGS THAT SLOW THE COURSE OF ARTHRITIS

Some drugs don't work just on symptoms—stiffness and pain; they actually work on the arthritis itself, slowing the rate at which the disease progresses. Doctors call these DMARDs (disease-modifying anti-rheumatic drugs).

Unfortunately, to date no drugs have been approved for slowing the rate of osteoarthritis. The only substances thought by some to potentially modify the course of that disease are called *glucosamine* and *chondroitin,* which are available in supplements. But how effective they are is controversial. Glucosamine and chondroitin are discussed in greater detail in Chapter 9.

The good news, at least for people with rheumatoid arthritis and other types of inflammatory arthritis, is that there are about a dozen drugs that can help slow the rate of joint deterioration. Often, doctors will prescribe two or three of them in combination. We divide these medications into two categories: "Easy on the Body" and "Hard on the Body."

Easy on the body

Side effects with these drugs are rare and, if they do occur, are generally mild. These medications tend to be most effective in patients whose arthritis is not too advanced.

BRAND NAME: Arava

GENERIC NAME: leflunomide

BEST CANDIDATE: rheumatoid arthritis

COST PER 30 DAYS: $$$$$

NOTES: Approved for use in the United States since 1999, leflunomide interferes with the replication of white blood cells, which multiply faster than other cells and thereby hasten the progression of the disease. The drug starts working within 3–6 weeks and is usually well tolerated, although blood counts and tests for liver function should be checked every 1–3 months. The main side effect appears to be diarrhea. If that occurs, a drug called *cholestyramine* is administered to draw the leflunomide out of the body. Otherwise, it can remain in the body causing problems for up to 2 years. Women should not take this drug if they are pregnant or trying to become pregnant.

BRAND NAME: Azulfidine

GENERIC NAME: sulfasalazine

BEST CANDIDATE: spondyloarthritis and rheumatoid arthritis

COST PER 30 DAYS: $

NOTES: Half aspirin and half antibiotic, this medication helps slow the course of not just rheumatoid arthritis but also ankylosing spondylitis, Reiter's syndrome, and other inflammatory forms of arthritis. It's generally well tolerated, although it may cause some mild stomach upset in the form of bloating or diarrhea. Blood tests for liver function should be conducted every 1–3 months to check for blood count suppression. Women should not take this drug if they are pregnant or trying to become pregnant.

BRAND NAME: Minocin, Dynacin, and others

GENERIC NAME: minocycline

BEST CANDIDATE: mild rheumatoid arthritis

COST PER 30 DAYS: $

NOTES: Like auranofin (see the following page), this medication falls somewhere between a symptom reliever and a disease retardant. It gained favor in the 1970s when a doctor in Washington prescribed it for a group of senators' wives with arthritis, even though it had not been proven effective in clinical trials. The wives were so impressed with the results that they talked their husbands into forcing the National Institutes of Health to appropriate funds for minocycline research. Lo and behold, the drug proved better than placebo for improving arthritis symptoms (but it never definitively was shown to stem joint erosion). Women should not take this drug if they are pregnant or trying to become pregnant. Children should not take it either—it is a tetracycline, which can permanently stain teeth.

BRAND NAME: Plaquenil

GENERIC NAME: hydroxychloroquine

BEST CANDIDATE: rheumatoid arthritis, Sjögren's syndrome, or lupus

COST PER 30 DAYS: $$$

NOTES: Plaquenil is actually an antimalarial drug. The benefit of antimalarials for people with arthritis was accidentally discovered in the 1950s, when it was noticed that people with rheumatoid arthritis who took those medications in preparation for travel to Africa experienced a decrease in arthritis symptoms. The main side effect is progressive loss of vision—the drug can build up in the retina and block the optic nerve—but it's completely preventable as long as you are examined by an ophthalmologist every 6 months. He or she can see the problem taking shape before there's any serious damage, and as long as you discontinue the medication (should that be advised), your vision will remain intact. Other possible side effects include nausea, rash, or a bitter taste in the mouth. Women should not take this drug if they are pregnant or trying to become pregnant.

BRAND NAME: Ridaura

GENERIC NAME: auranofin

BEST CANDIDATE: mild rheumatoid arthritis

COST PER 30 DAYS: $$$$

NOTES: This drug, part of which is actually the chemical element gold, falls somewhere between the category of slowing the course of arthritis and simply relieving symptoms. It reduces inflammation but doesn't necessarily keep joints from getting "chewed up." Nonetheless, it has a role in treating mild arthritis. (It's probably not going to help people whose disease is progressing aggressively.) Its only major side effect is diarrhea, which can often be prevented with the simple step of adopting a high-fiber diet. Women should not take this drug if they are pregnant or trying to become pregnant.

Hard on the Body

These drugs are usually reserved for people whose arthritis is very advanced or very severe. They tend to come with more serious side effects.

BRAND NAME: Cytoxan

GENERIC NAME: cyclophosphamide

BEST CANDIDATE: those for whom nothing else works—it increases the risk for certain cancers, namely bladder cancer, leukemia, and lymphoma

COST PER 30 DAYS: $$ (given orally); $$$$$ (given intravenously)

NOTES: Besides increasing cancer risk, it can cause immune suppression (which may lead to infections). In addition, it can suppress red blood cell production, paving the way for anemia. It can also decrease blood platelet production, which increases the risk for excess bleeding. Blood-test monitoring is required monthly, or even more often in some cases. Women should not take this drug if they are pregnant or trying to become pregnant. With prolonged use, it will sterilize women (and, rarely, men).

BRAND NAME: Imuran

GENERIC NAME: azathioprine

BEST CANDIDATE: lupus and severe rheumatoid arthritis

COST PER 30 DAYS: $$$

NOTES: This mainstay drug for kidney transplants is not used much anymore for arthritic diseases because it increases the risk for infection. It can also cause diarrhea, rashes, and inflammation of the pancreas, an organ that's crucial to the proper digestion of foods. Blood tests are required every 1–3 months to check the state of the white blood cells. Women should not take this drug if they are pregnant or trying to become pregnant, except on a doctor's direct recommendation.

BRAND NAME(S): Myochrysine, Solganal

GENERIC NAME: gold

BEST CANDIDATE: rheumatoid arthritis

TYPICAL DAILY DOSE: Injected intramuscularly rather than taken by mouth. Injections are weekly for the first 4–6 months (which means a weekly visit to the doctor's office). After that time (it takes that long to see whether there's a response), the injections can be cut back to every other week, then to every third week, and even to once a month if the symptoms remain under control.

COST PER 30 DAYS: $$$$$ (cost includes weekly monitoring)

NOTES: This drug, the first ever shown to prevent joint damage in rheumatoid arthritis back in the early 1960s, is literally gold (and much more potent than Ridaura, gold taken orally). Before each injection, the doctor takes urine and blood samples to check for gold's side effects: kidney inflammation, reduced ability to fight infections, and aplastic anemia, which is a serious decrease in red blood cell production. Women should not take this drug if they are pregnant or trying to become pregnant.

BRAND NAME: Rheumatrex

GENERIC NAME: methotrexate

BEST CANDIDATE: moderate to severe rheumatoid arthritis, psoriatic arthritis, sometimes lupus and vasculitis

COST PER 30 DAYS: $$

NOTES: This drug, taken by mouth *or* administered by intramuscular injection, has revolutionized the care of rheumatoid arthritis and psoriatic arthritis. People are often afraid of it because it's a cancer drug used to treat leukemia. But the dose used to kill cancer cells is on the order of 1,000 milligrams at a time. At the very low doses given for arthritis (5–30 mg once a week), it doesn't kill cells. It simply suppresses inflammation. The main risks that come with taking methotrexate are liver-related cirrhosis and hepatitis. Blood tests for liver function are required every 1–3 months. In addition, absolutely no alcoholic beverages are permitted, as they increase the risk for liver problems. A much more rare complication is an allergic reaction in the lungs, which can be life-threatening. Symptoms are a lot like those of pneumonia and include fever, cough, and abnormal chest X-rays. Treatment often requires hospitalization. Women should not take this drug if they are pregnant or trying to become pregnant (see the box below).

If you're pregnant . . .

The arthritis drug methotrexate causes stillbirths and birth defects comparable to those caused by thalidomide—the drug that caused children to be born with finlike arms back in the 1960s. A pregnant woman should *never* take it, nor should a woman become pregnant while taking it. The drug is so potent that even a man taking it should not impregnate a woman. The same goes for Arava. It is okay for potential fathers to take the other drugs listed above, even though they are not safe for expectant or soon-to-be-expectant mothers.

BRAND NAME(S): Sandimmune, Neoral

GENERIC NAME: cyclosporin

BEST CANDIDATE: those whose arthritis is hard to control with other medications

COST PER 30 DAYS: $$$$$

NOTES: This is the drug that made organ transplants possible; it helps prevent organ rejection by suppressing the body's immune response to foreign bodies. Likewise, it suppresses the autoimmune process that advances arthritis. Unfortunately, it comes with several potential down sides. These include kidney dysfunction (which has to be watched quite closely), elevated blood pressure, suppression of white blood cells to the point of increasing the risk for developing infections, and hirsutism—primarily facial hair—even in women.

Two other drugs just approved in 2000, Enbrel (etanercept) and Remicade (infliximab), are part of a growing class of arthritis drugs that appear to be the most effective against the disease to date. (A third drug, Anakinra, was just approved as we went to press.) Their effectiveness is due in part to the fact that they are the most specifically targeted drugs we have for treating rheumatoid arthritis. They are not cancer drugs or organ transplant drugs.

They work to suppress the immune system in a very particular way. Specifically, they inhibit the action of "messenger" proteins in the body, called *cytokines,* which white cells use to "communicate" among themselves. Once the white cells "lose touch" with each other, they lose their ability to mount an attack on joints.

BRAND NAME: Enbrel

GENERIC NAME: etanercept

BEST CANDIDATE: severe rheumatoid arthritis not responding to oral medications

DELIVERY MECHANISM: injections twice a week under the skin (most people can learn to inject themselves)

COST PER 30 DAYS: $$$$$

NOTES: The main risk is an increased chance of infections because it suppresses the immune system. For that reason, anyone taking Enbrel must be certain to get a flu shot every year. It's also important to get

Physically removing arthritis-causing compounds from the body

Imagine a machine that could actually filter from the body the antibodies that set white cells into motion and thereby accelerate joint damage. There is one. It's called Prosorba, and it works in much the same way that a dialysis machine works to filter waste from the body when the kidneys no longer can. Prosorba patients are hooked up to the machine once a week for 12 weeks, 2 hours per session. (Not all hospitals have it.) It generally takes at least six treatments to see results, during which time you can get flulike symptoms such as chills and fever.

Common adverse effects include transiently worsening joint pain and fatigue, although these tend to last only for a day or two after each treatment. The bigger problem is that only about one in three patients respond to the treatment, which is why doctors tend to use it only when drugs have failed.

checked out by your doctor if you get a fever or cold that lasts more than a few days or is especially severe. You will also need to undergo periodic blood tests. Women should not take this drug if they are pregnant or trying to become pregnant.

BRAND NAME: Remicade

GENERIC NAME: infliximab

BEST CANDIDATE: severe rheumatoid arthritis not responding to oral medications

DELIVERY MECHANISM: intravenous injections every 6 weeks (after an initial startup of three IVs over a 6-week period)

COST PER 30 DAYS: $$$$$

NOTES: Similar to Enbrel, the main risk is an increased chance of infections because it suppresses the immune system. For that reason, anyone taking Remicade must be certain to get a flu shot every year. It's also important to get checked out by your doctor if you get a fever or cold that lasts more than a few days or is especially severe. You will also need to undergo periodic blood tests. Women should not take this drug if they are pregnant or trying to become pregnant.

It is important that you talk with your doctor about medications and that your doctor knows your entire medical history so that he or she can guide you in the safest, most effective manner. There is no doubt that over the next few years there will be new medications approved to help with arthritis. But remember that no medication alone will help you climb mountains, play tennis, or garden for hours. Your body needs the stimulus of exercise and the right nutrients from your diet to fight arthritis best—but medications can make all the difference in those efforts.

CHAPTER 8

The Ins and Outs of Joint Replacement Surgery

■

I had been having trouble with my left knee for years," says Sister Mary Patrice, age 71. "But the exercises that Kristin taught me to do were wonderful. I could walk so much better, and with much less pain. Then, about a year ago, I came down with a terrible, terrible cold. I was coming down the stairs at school [Sister Mary Patrice is the dean of discipline at a Catholic high school], and I missed the bottom step and came down on both knees. After that I couldn't put *any* weight on the bad one. I never really wanted to have surgery, but I went to see the orthopedic surgeon."

Sixty-year-old Earl, a lieutenant firefighter, developed osteoarthritis in his left hip in his mid-fifties. "I was coming down the pole, responding to a fire," he says. "Someone had removed the pad at the bottom. I landed on my tailbone and was laid up for about 4 months. At first I had recurring pain in my back, but then I started getting some burning in my hip, a tightness there when I bent down to tie my shoes. The pain was a 'two' or 'three' for the first few years. Then I wasn't able to get my ankle up to my knee to put on a sock or tie my shoe. The pain went anywhere from a 'five' to an 'eight.' The Vioxx I was taking alleviated the pain, so it was tolerable, but it wasn't making me mobile. Then my primary care physician recommended that I go see an orthopedic surgeon. The surgeon didn't recommend surgery right away— not until I had a problem sleeping at night. No matter what position I was in, it ached. Even sitting—it hurt without any movement."

Sometimes, despite doing everything you can to keep your arthritis under control, you simply can no longer find relief from pain. Or maybe you're reading this book years after your pain began, so the joint deterioration has already progressed to the point that making lifestyle changes simply is not going to be enough to keep pain under control. Whatever the reason, if pain is unrelenting, it's time to consider joint replacement surgery, known in medical circles as *arthroplasty.*

That may seem like a drastic solution, but rest assured that if you undergo surgery to replace a joint that's too far gone, you're not alone. The ability to replace worn-away joints has revolutionized arthritis care in the last two decades, and literally hundreds of thousands of Americans undergo joint replacement every year. Some 245,000 knee replacements are performed annually in the United States alone, as well as 137,000 hip replacements!

And the relief from pain is *dramatic.* Says Earl, "The relief from the hip pain was immediate. I had some surgery pain at first. But it was a *lot* less pain than the hip had been causing. The day I was operated on they had me up with a walker. I was walking without the walker within 3 days."

Sister Mary Patrice tells a similar story. "Even the second or third day after the surgery, I could walk to the bathroom."

The relief from pain and the improvement in mobility makes sense. Once you've lost so much cartilage that bone is sitting directly on top of bone, you've got a carpentry problem—and need a carpentry solution. Until there is a procedure that grows back cartilage, surgery is the only answer.

ARE YOU A SURGERY CANDIDATE?

There are four conditions, any one of which is reason enough to consider arthritis surgery:

- pain that hasn't responded to nonsurgical treatment
- unbearable pain at rest
- unbearable pain at night
- inability to function because the joint doesn't move properly, even if there is not much pain

If any of those describes your condition, you should speak to your physician about the advisability of seeking joint replacement. Of course, it's important to be in good-enough overall health to undergo the general (or spinal) anesthesia required for the operation. If you have heart disease, high blood pressure, a history of stroke, emphysema, cancer, or some other illness, you are at higher risk for complications. That doesn't necessarily mean that you should live with pain for the rest of your life. But your primary care physician and your orthopedist should discuss with you the risks and benefits of surgery. Your doctors may decide that you should undergo additional testing to assess just how great your risk is. You might need a stress test (treadmill test), lung-function tests, an echocardiogram (ultrasound of your heart and or carotid arteries), or even a cardiac catheterization (X-rays of your coronary arteries to look for blockages) before you can have a joint replaced. At each step, you and your physicians will need to decide if the additional risk is worth it. If it is, go on. If you decide that your risk is quite high and that surgery is not a reasonable option, at least you will have made an informed choice.

Are exercise and nutrition of any benefit?

Does opting for surgery at some point mean that going through our exercise and dietary program was for naught? Not at all! If you've made an effort to help your joints beforehand, the better your body will be able to handle the new, artificial joint afterward. For instance, if you've strengthened the muscles surrounding your joint with strength training, there will be less stress on the new joint once it's put in. The joint will be much better protected when you're up and around again. Indeed, how much muscle you have before surgery is a strong predictor of how well you're going to do after surgery.

Following our targeted exercise program can also *delay* surgery as long as possible in people who eventually need it. An artificial joint works at its peak capacity for 10–15 years—in some cases longer than 20 years. So the later in life you have the surgery, the less the chance that you'll need to have it again. That's particularly important in light of the fact that it's harder for the surgery to go as smoothly the second time around. Once bone surrounding the joint has already been manipulated to accommodate a prosthesis, or artificial joint, it scars and is harder to manipulate again.

That said, it should be noted that most people delay surgery *too* long, as Ronenn has found in his practice. "A lot of what I do is try to convince patients to have the surgery," he comments. "People are afraid of surgery, and they put it off even when their pain has gotten to the point where it's the logical solution." Of course, the longer the pain goes on, the more deconditioned the muscles around the joint get, and the harder it is to recover strength in the joint after the operation.

Have reasonable expectations

Surgery has dramatic effects in the vast majority of cases. Even with the comments from Sister Mary Patrice and Earl, we can't emphasize enough the relief from pain that most people feel when they replace a joint in the hip, knee, shoulder, or other area of the body. However, life after joint replacement, while usually pain free, is not exactly the same as life before the pain of

Too few women opting for hip and knee replacements

When The Arthritis Foundation polled 2,000 people for their views on pain, six in ten said it was "just something you have to live with." But that's simply not the case, especially when it comes to arthritis pain. Joint replacement surgery can completely eradicate hip, knee, or other joint pain that has proven debilitating for years.

Women are less likely than men to take advantage of surgery to relieve unrelenting arthritis pain. According to a Canadian study of people 55 and older, the underuse of *arthroplasty*, or joint replacement, is three times greater in women than in men. It is not entirely clear why. It could be that their primary care physicians are not referring them to orthopedic surgeons as routinely. Or maybe women are less inclined to opt for surgery because they have a higher pain threshold or more worries about who's going to care for their loved ones while they recover from the operation.

Whatever the reason, Ronenn comments that many women—and men—once they have the surgery, come back to him and say, "Why did I wait so long?"

arthritis set in. That is, there are some things surgery *can't* do, and it's important to be realistic.

For instance, surgery won't give you 100 percent of the range of motion your hip had when you were 20 years old. Depending on your own particular anatomy, you may regain anywhere from half to two-thirds or even more of your range of motion. But by the same token, you may not be able to tie your shoes without some contortions or even without some assistance, say, from a long shoehorn or even another person. You certainly won't be able to engage in high-impact sports like running, jogging, tennis, basketball, and the like. Such activities will pound your new hip and could cause it to fail prematurely.

But—and this is a big "but"—while the return of joint function isn't complete, *the loss of joint motion usually affects people much less than constant pain does,* and there will be much you can do that you might not have been able to do for some time. Activities like swimming and playing golf will come easily, as will riding a bike or taking walks. Even more important, day-to-day activities that may have been causing extreme discomfort, such as climbing stairs or getting out of a chair, will be easy again. Only about 5 percent of people who undergo joint replacement surgery do not experience significant improvements.

How to prepare for the operation

As with any surgery, a physical exam before arthroplasty will be required to make sure your body is up to the operation. The doctor will check your heart function as well as the functioning of other body organs. You will also need to give samples of blood and urine for various diagnostic tests. You should visit the dentist beforehand, too. Untreated cavities could make you more prone to infection.

Note that you may be asked to donate your own blood in advance, to be given back to you at the time of surgery. This is by far the safest way to get blood (you can't get infected by or be allergic to your own blood!), so if your doctor recommends this, you should definitely agree to it.

If you take nonsteroidal anti-inflammatories (NSAIDs) you will be told to discontinue them about a week before the surgery (sometimes longer, depending on the situation), as they can make you more prone to bleed excessively during the operation. Acetaminophen (Tylenol) may be safely taken instead.

Are you having the wrong operation?

If you are very overweight (BMI over 40, see pages 42–43) and have knee or hip osteoarthritis, consider whether a different operation may be the one you really need. In many cases surgery for weight loss (intestinal bypass) can cause so much needed weight loss that knee and hip pain disappears—and you'll be much healthier in other ways, too! This is especially true for individuals who are 50 years of age or younger. Most artificial joints don't last more than 20 years; the operations are hard to perform on very overweight individuals; and the doctor is only treating the symptom (joint pain), not the root of the problem (excess body weight).

If you are overweight, it's a good idea to try to lose some excess pounds before the surgery. Obese people, in particular, often have a harder time after the operation. Extra folds of tissue that are hard to keep dry and clean increase the chance of infection at the incision site. It's also harder to control blood loss through several inches of fat. Some surgeons will not even operate on people above a certain weight.

You should also take some presurgery precautions to make sure the several weeks of recuperation will be as easy as possible once you return home. The American Academy of Orthopaedic Surgeons recommends a number of steps so that your home will be "rehab-friendly," particularly if you're going for hip joint replacement. Many of these steps require the use of items like shower benches and dressing sticks. Ask your surgeon or his or her office staff about how to find these items, several of which can be bought or rented from your physical therapist while you are in the hospital.

- Put handrails along all stairways.
- Make sure you have a stable chair for your early recovery. It should have a firm seat cushion that allows your knees to remain lower than your hips, a firm back, and two arms.
- Obtain a raised toilet seat.

- Get a stable shower bench or chair for bathing.
- Get a long-handled sponge and shower hose.
- Get a dressing stick, a sock aid, and a long-handled shoe horn for putting on and taking off shoes and socks without excessively bending your new hip.
- Have on hand a "reacher" that will allow you to grab objects without excessive bending of your hips.
- Buy firm pillows to sit on that keep your knees lower than your hips while sitting on chairs, sofas, and in the car.
- Remove all loose carpets and electrical cords from areas where you walk in your home.
- Make sure you have sturdy, comfortable shoes.

THE SURGERY ITSELF

The operation itself, which is basically the same whether you're replacing a joint because of osteoarthritis or rheumatoid arthritis, is not a terribly complicated procedure as far as operations go. First, the anesthesia team will discuss which type of anesthesia is best for you. The most common types for joint replacement surgery are general anesthesia (which puts you to sleep throughout the procedure) and spinal anesthesia (which allows you to be awake but anesthetizes your body from the waist down).

The actual surgical procedure takes a few hours. First, an orthopedic surgeon cuts out whatever's left of the damaged joint cartilage along with some bone on either side of it. Then he or she restores joint alignment and function with artificial parts. Many different designs and materials are currently used, but all consist of two basic components:

- the socket component (a durable plastic cup for hip and shoulder, and a saucer shape for the knee), which may have an outer metal shell
- the ball component, or joint (made of a very smooth metal)

For a hip replacement, the surgeon anchors the socket in the pelvis and then proceeds to push the ball right into the space that has been carved out of the thigh bone. For a knee replacement, the ends of the femur (thigh bone) and tibia (leg bone) are sawed off, and artificial parts are tapped into place at the newly exposed ends of the bones. Sometimes special surgical cement is used to fill the gap between the prosthesis, or artificial joint, and the remaining natural bone in order to secure the new hardware. A non-cemented prosthesis has also been developed for use in younger, more active patients. Your surgeon will recommend which system to use depending on your situation.

After surgery you will be moved to the recovery room, where you will re-main for a few hours while your "coming out of" the anesthesia is moni-tored. After you awaken fully, you will be taken to your hospital room.

During the healing process, which takes place over several months, the body's bone naturally grows around the prosthetic joint, truly allowing it to become integrated in place of the old, damaged joint. You'll generally be home from the hospital within 3–4 days.

WHAT TO EXPECT POSTOPERATIVELY

Immediately after the operation, arthritis pain that may have been debilitat-ing you for years will be gone. There will, however, be pain from the incision, which lasts 1–2 weeks. Fortunately, narcotics like percocet, Percodan, oxy-codone, or Dilaudid are prescribed to dull the discomfort.

Better still, complications from joint replacement surgery are uncom-mon. Infections in the wound occur in fewer than 2 percent of cases. Com-plications of anesthesia, such as heart attack or stroke, are even less common. The most common complication is *venous thrombosis,* a blood clot in the leg that causes leg pain and swelling. More important, a piece of the clot can break off and travel through the bloodstream to lodge in the lung, a danger-ous and sometimes fatal situation called a *pulmonary embolus.* But such in-stances are rare, in large part because doctors often prescribe blood thinners for the first month or two after surgery in order to prevent these clots.

Starting physical therapy

Once you're home, you're going to have to learn to walk again with the help of a physical therapist, assuming the joint replacement is in the hip or knee.

How to interview your surgeon

The way health care is dispensed in the United States, most of the time the orthopedic surgeon who conducts your arthroplasty will be chosen by your doctor or by your health-insurance provider. But you may very well have at least some choice in the matter. If you do, there are three important questions to ask a prospective surgeon, four if you have rheumatoid arthritis (and don't be shy about asking them!):

1. How many operations of this type have you done? (More than a hundred is a good number.)
2. What's your success rate? (It should be above 80 percent altogether. Five years after the operation, 90 percent of patients should still be pain free; 10 years after, 80–85 percent should be pain free.)
3. Where did you do your orthopedic training? (An orthopedic surgeon who has trained at a reputable hospital is a good bet.)
4. (For those who have rheumatoid arthritis): Do you have experience operating on people with rheumatoid arthritis as opposed to osteoarthritis? Joint replacement in someone who has rheumatoid arthritis tends to be more complicated than in someone with osteoarthritis because there's often more tissue destruction. And the tissue that's there is much more fragile, more easily "broken." In addition, while someone who usually operates on osteoarthritis patients might only have experience replacing joints in the knees or hip, someone with rheumatoid arthritis might need surgery to replace a joint in, say, a knuckle, elbow, or wrist.

Truth be told, many surgeons don't have the best bedside manner. If the surgeon you see responds to these questions in a gruff or even a sharp manner, don't be too surprised. Moreover, don't assume he or she is not the best person for the job—you need the surgeon's technical skills, not friendship. Feeling comfortable with the doctor's personality isn't as important as it is with your primary care physician.

Of course, in any case, check with your state board of medical licensure and ask whether the surgeon has had any complaints, lawsuits, or reprimands against him or her. It's public information, and many states allow you to check this on their websites. Even if a doctor has been sued once or even more, that does not mean that he or she is not competent. Today, every doctor expects to get sued at least once, and most suits are dismissed or decided in favor of the doctor. But a pattern of recurrent complaints and suits suggests someone to avoid. Each state's medical board is listed in the "Government" section of the white pages and is used to dealing with consumer questions.

The Orthopaedic Academy agrees that "exercise is a critical component of home care, particularly during the first few weeks after surgery."

For the first couple of weeks, you'll get around with a walker or crutches. The idea is to let the new joint come together with the surrounding bone without putting any stress on the area. Then, over the course of 6–8 weeks, you'll gradually put more weight on the joint, going from two crutches to one crutch, from one crutch to a cane, and so on. Everyone progresses through the various stages at his or her own pace, depending on such variables as pain threshold.

Whatever your pace, you will then begin a walking program, first in the house and later outside, which will slowly increase your stamina and mobility and enable you to bathe and engage in other activities of daily living independently. Your therapist will give you exercises to increase your range of motion in the new joint and may also have you use rubber bands to start building up your strength.

Once you can walk comfortably on a flat surface, stairs are next. You will be asked to do a series of exercises to maximize the range of motion in your new hip (or other joint) every day, and you'll be able to resume most normal activities of daily living in 3–6 weeks.

Once the physical therapy sequence has been completed—after 6 weeks or so—you will be ready for more intense activities, but you should never subject your replaced joint to any high-impact exercise such as jogging, basketball, football, soccer, etc. However, as we said earlier, golfing is fine, as are gardening, walking, swimming, and most other enjoyable activities!

Toward the latter stages of rehabilitation, when you're more or less walking like your old self, you should also restart (or start) our strength-training program. The better the shape of the muscles supporting your new joint, the better the joint will be able to work—and the longer it will last. Talk to your doctor or therapist about when it is appropriate to start our program and if any particular modifications need to be made.

Don't be afraid to take the plunge if necessary

Again, we can't emphasize enough that if you are in pain that cannot be quelled, a discussion with your doctor about joint replacement surgery is in order. As Sister Mary Patrice comments, "Before the surgery, I thought, 'What's the use? I'll be eighty in ten years.' But now I feel wonderful. I really do. I can zip along corridors, get up and down off a stool, get up stairs. I have more energy throughout the day."

As for Earl, he says that "right now I can do just about anything I want—gardening, hunting, fishing. I'm a physical person as far as working around the yard and things like that. Now I can go for a walk again without being in excruciating pain. Just this week my wife and I put up strapping for the porch roof on our vacation home.

"Anybody you know who's going through that aggravation—get it done," he advises. "There's nothing to be afraid of. I'm very happy with the outcome."

CHAPTER 9

Complementary Approaches

◼

I was desperate enough to the point where I'd try just about anything," says Fred, a 37-year-old medical school researcher. He had been suffering from osteoarthritis of the hip since he was 27, tracing it back to his college football days as an offensive lineman. Six feet, 3 inches tall, Fred had weighed 260 pounds in school. That's a lot of pressure on the hip as a body runs, jumps, and falls in a tackle.

The pain had gotten to the point, says Fred, "where I was thinking about it all the time. It was hard to sleep—a combination of burning and inflammation combined with a dull ache."

Then he started taking supplements of glucosamine and chondroitin, which some studies suggest may help relieve arthritis pain. "Whether the difference was real or perceived," Fred comments, "I felt much better. I was pretty much sold on it. Within 3 weeks I was able to go from not being able to do *any* exercise to working out on an elliptical trainer or stationary bike.

"No question it has changed the quality of my life. I had been resigned to the fact that I had a pretty limited lifestyle to look forward to, especially since I was pretty far, age-wise, from being a candidate for hip replacement."

Forty-year-old Mark tells a different story. He, too, has osteoarthritis of the hip, saying that "it probably started from an injury I had when I fell off the back of a motorcycle at sixteen." And he, too, took a combination glucosamine/chondroitin supplement—for about 8 months. However, Mark "found that it really had no effect on my hip." He still rides a bike four or five times a week but says he has to use a prescription anti-inflammatory drug for anything that stresses his hip more than that.

Fred and Mark are not alone in trying out unconventional therapies. Desperate to seek more relief from their pain and immobility than traditional medicine is sometimes able to offer, most people with arthritis turn to treatments that are outside the purview of what their doctors recommend. These include a wide range of things: yoga, strict vegetarian diets, meditation, herbs, acupuncture, copper bracelets, bee stings, topical ointments, and the list goes on.

In many cases, very little is known about these nontraditional approaches. One reason is that with arthritis, rheumatoid arthritis in particular, the illness flares and subsides without any discernible pattern, so sometimes it might seem as though a treatment is working when it's simply the disease taking its natural course and is in a "dormant" period for a while.

Then, too, a lot of studies on unconventional treatments are not conducted as rigorously as studies for treatments that have made their way into mainstream medicine. Drugs approved by the Food and Drug Administration for doctors to prescribe have been through gold-standard studies known as placebo-controlled trials. That means that while some of the volunteers get the real thing, some get a placebo, or dummy pill. That's really important because even in the best of studies, up to 30 percent of those in the placebo group end up feeling better. If 30 percent of those who get the actual treatment also feel better, then you know that a treatment that *appears* to be relieving pain is really no more effective than a sugar pill. The treatment (drug) under study has to perform significantly better than the placebo to be considered an effective treatment.

You might ask, "What's the difference as long as the person is in less pain?" Well, the difference could be a lot of money wasted on an expensive product that isn't doing any more than a sugar cube would. Furthermore, a trial with a placebo group will yield valuable information about any potential side effects of a particular treatment that differ from the side effects some people perceive with placebos—what they are, how severe they can get, and whether they're reversible. That's crucial, because even if a treatment turns out to be ineffective, it can still interfere with metabolism and cause harm.

What it all comes down to is that you need to be careful about trying complementary therapies. Don't believe everything you're told, especially from those who will profit from your purchase of a treatment. While there are some promising complementary therapies out there, many have not been investigated at all.

That said, however, many physicians are becoming more supportive of their patients trying various unconventional therapies despite the lack of solid evidence. After all, they want their patients to feel better, and, if something appears to be helping relieve pain and stiffness—or at least not hurting—doctors don't want to stand in their way.

That's what this chapter is all about—separating out the promising complementary therapies from the useless, and sometimes harmful, ones. Of course, it is beyond the scope of this book to tell you everything about every single complementary treatment available. But here we have provided background information on a number of the more popular complementary approaches, including whether there is any solid research to back up claims and whether there are any safety issues.

Should you decide to try one or more of these approaches, you might be inclined not to tell your doctor for fear that he or she will pooh-pooh your decision or try to talk you out of it. That's not a good idea. You should always let your physician know if you are engaged in any complementary practices because that way he or she can take what you're doing into consideration and adjust your treatment as necessary. For instance, if you decide to take a particular herb, the doctor can provide guidelines for safety, such as potential dangerous interactions with your current drugs. If you follow an unusual diet, your physician may recommend certain nutrition supplements. In addition, certain therapies people use to quell arthritis pain have actually been shown to be harmful, and your doctor can steer you away from something that could worsen your health.

Of course, just as with conventional drugs, some complementary therapies turn out to be more beneficial for some people than for others (which may be at least part of the reason that Fred and Mark had different experiences with glucosamine/chondroitin supplements). Thus, a bit of trial and error, just like with prescription drugs, might be in order.

Herewith, a guide to what might work, and apparently has worked for some people, as well as a guide to what's known to be useless or, worse, will waste your time, money, and emotional energy in the process.

The complementary therapies listed below (in alphabetical order) are divided into three categories: Things You Swallow; Things You Apply (or Wear); and Things You Do (or Have Done *to* You). In each case we'll provide the mechanism for how it's proposed to work (if there is one); proof of efficacy—or lack thereof; safety issues; and any other information that's germane to the particular therapy. Take a look, too, at the "Resources" section at the back of the book for additional information. We especially encourage you to read The Arthritis Foundation's *Guide to Alternative Therapies* (see "Resources" for a full reference), an excellent book that goes into great detail about many types of alternative therapies.

Note: We don't advocate using unconventional treatments *in place of* traditional medical treatment, which often means trading tested remedies for unproven therapies. On the other hand, using these treatments *in conjunction with* traditional medical approaches is considered complementary medicine—the safest and most beneficial approach.

THINGS YOU SWALLOW

Cartilage (shark, cow, and chicken)

Since arthritis causes loss of cartilage from joints, it is attractive to think that eating cartilage could reverse this effect. That, in part, is what has led to the popularity of cartilage supplements, which are made from sharks, cows (bovine), and chickens.

How it's said to work: Using cartilage medicinally began in the early 1950s, when cow cartilage was found to promote the healing of wounds. And dried, pulverized shark cartilage has been studied as an inhibitor of tumor growth. As far as treating arthritis symptoms, it has been said that cartilage is beneficial in reducing inflammation.

Proof: We know of not a single clinical trial demonstrating the ability of shark, cow, or chicken cartilage to mitigate arthritis symptoms. However, there is evidence from a number of trials that collagen II, which can be extracted from cartilage, is beneficial for people with rheumatoid arthritis. Several well-controlled studies have shown that collagen II extract at low doses—around 60 micrograms per day—has a modest effect in lessening joint tenderness and swelling. More research is under way that will further expand our knowledge of the effects of collagen II on rheumatoid arthritis.

Safety issues: Cartilage at high doses can cause nausea. Also, if you use collagen II, talk to your doctor about obtaining a pure source, and take only small doses. Collagen II is not readily available over the counter, but it can be bought over the Internet.

The bottom line: There is good evidence that taking shark, cow, or chicken cartilage has *no* effect on arthritis. If you have rheumatoid arthritis, there is some evidence that taking small doses of collagen II may relieve symptoms to a mild degree.

Chinese herbs

Chinese herbal medicine has been practiced for more than 4,000 years. The thinking of those who practice it is that the solution to ailments is found by reaching a balance between the two energies contained in everything that has life: yin and yang. The interactions of these energies produce Qi (pronounced *chee*), or life force, and illnesses and their symptoms are described in terms of how yin, yang, and Qi are out of kilter and affect the workings of various organs and bodily functions.

How it's said to work: Arthritis, in particular, is described as an *obstruction* of Qi, and different combinations of herbs with yin or yang properties are used to correct the imbalance that leads to the obstruction and set things right. Different herbs are used depending on the symptoms. There are hundreds of Chinese herbs purported to reduce pain, to lessen swelling, to control stiffness, or combinations thereof. When we went to one Chinese herb website and did a search for Chinese herbs used to treat arthritis, we came up with almost a hundred herb or herb combinations there alone, from Du Huo, Zhi Gan Cao, and Bai Shao to *tripterygium wilfordii,* to name a few.

Proof: Most information on Chinese herbs has come from uncontrolled trials. In fact, there have been few clinical trials published in well-respected English-language journals. Most have been published only in Chinese journals and have never been translated, so they are difficult for most U.S. arthritis researchers to interpret. However, the sheer number of reports is impressive, with some intriguing results.

Some test-tube research, for instance, has suggested that the herb *triptery-gium wilfordii* (thunder god vine) may have immunosuppressive properties—a plus if you want to control swelling and inflammation. And in one controlled human study, patients with rheumatoid arthritis who took herbs reported significant improvement in symptoms as well as blood tests over a period of 12 weeks. An *un*controlled study suggested that treatment with herbs "cured" or at least markedly improved symptoms in 20 out of 34 people with rheumatoid arthritis. But because there was no placebo group, it is difficult to interpret these results.

Safety issues: Because of the lack of well-controlled research, we urge you to consider Chinese herbs with caution—particularly since they are not subject to premarket safety testing and can contain harmful adulterants. If you decide to try Chinese herbs, talk with your doctor first, as many could interfere with medications you are taking—or worsen other conditions you may have. The Food and Drug Administration has taken several Chinese herbs off the U.S. market in recent years because of unexpected side effects, including cancers and deaths.

The bottom line: There is no solid evidence to suggest that Chinese herbs either help or hinder arthritis, so if you decide to try them, do so for several months and then reassess whether they are helpful. *Always* consult your physician about adding herbs to your current treatment. Even better would be to ask your doctor to work on your case in conjunction with a qualified Oriental medicine practitioner. The American Association of Oriental Medicine (AAOM), whose members are regarded as the most highly qualified to use Chinese herbs and other Asian remedies in the United States, has a national referral list for Oriental medicine practitioners who are board-certified by that organization. (See "Resources" for more information.)

Chondroitin/glucosamine

Both chondroitin and glucosamine are normal components of cartilage, specifically of the proteoglycans in the cartilage. There is a constant turnover of proteoglycans and collagen in a healthy joint, and this turnover is off balance in arthritis, with more destruction than construction.

How it's said to work: Ingestion of glucosamine and chondroitin may affect the metabolism of proteoglycans in the joint, decreasing destruction and increasing their construction. In addition, these substances may have some anti-inflammatory properties, decreasing the production of inflammatory products of the immune system. But the reality is that scientists don't really know yet why glucosamine and chondroitin seem to help.

Proof: It's not clear yet whether chondroitin and glucosamine do what they're purported to. When researchers at the Boston University Arthritis Center looked at the combined results of fifteen different studies conducted between 1996 and 1999, they found small to moderate overall benefits for individuals with osteoarthritis. But most of the studies were small and not well controlled. There is one exception, however. Out of 212 people with knee arthritis in Belgium, those who took glucosamine ended up with fewer painful symptoms. For more definitive answers, the National Institutes of Health are sponsoring a large research trial on glucosamine and chondroitin, but results won't be available until 2004 or 2005.

Safety issues: Both chondroitin and gluocsamine appear to be safe. Virtually no side effects have been reported that were greater or more intense than side effects in placebo groups. But people taking glucosamine who have diabetes should have their blood sugar checked regularly. There is some suggestion from a few human and animal studies that glucosamine may affect insulin metabolism. And regular users of anticoagulants like aspirin or heparin should have their blood-clotting times checked if they take chondroitin; there's a chance it could alter blood-clotting activity. Finally, people with allergies to shellfish should note that glucosamine is made from crab, lobster, and shrimp shells. An allergic reaction is unlikely, but at least bring it up to your doctor and see what he or she thinks.

The bottom line: There is evidence to suggest that glucosamine and chondroitin are helpful for osteoarthritis. Most studies have used 1,500 milligrams a day for glucosamine and 1,200 milligrams for chondroitin. The cost is anywhere from $30–$60 a month—or more. If you haven't experienced relief within a couple of months, you're probably not going to and should stop taking them.

CMO

CMO, or *cetyl myristoleate,* is a type of fatty acid that is derived from cows.

How it's said to work: Ads for CMO state that it can boost your immune function to help your body fight all kinds of arthritis. But no real mechanism has been established.

Proof: The proof is scant. A single National Institutes of Health study in mice suggests that CMO is beneficial, but to date there have been no controlled human studies.

Safety issues: It is not known whether CMO is dangerous or safe. But what *is* dangerous is that some CMO manufacturers say the only way for people to get the full CMO benefit is to stop taking their prescribed arthritis medications. Some manufacturers also say that you should neither eat chocolate nor drink alcohol or caffeine-containing beverages while taking CMO, but why is anybody's guess.

The bottom line: There is no evidence to suggest that CMO helps or hinders arthritis. Because of some safety concerns, we advise against taking it.

Devil's claw

Devil's claw tablets are made from the root of a plant that's native to Africa and Madagascar.

How it's said to work: Devil's claw is sold in Europe as well as Canada as a digestive aid and an appetite stimulant, but it also has been used to treat pain. The root contains compounds that are thought to have pain-killing and anti-inflammatory properties.

Proof: Studies in both animals and humans have been inconsistent as far as demonstrating any anti-inflammatory effect, either for rheumatoid arthritis or osteoarthritis. One reason may be that stomach acid can inactivate some of the root's components. In the one well-controlled trial reported (which looked at people with lower back pain rather than at people with arthritis), those taking devil's claw had reductions in pain greater than those of a placebo group. These results suggest that devil's claw may have some pain-relieving properties—but not necessarily anti-inflammatory properties.

Safety issues: Devil's claw can affect the rhythm of the heart and therefore may be risky for those with heart conditions. Also, because it stimulates gastric secretions, it should not be taken by people with duodonal ulcers or gall-stones. Furthermore, it interacts with Coumadin (warfarin) and possibly other blood thinners and therefore can cause bleeding. Finally, devil's claw can stimulate the muscles of the uterine wall and therefore should not be taken during pregnancy.

The bottom line: There is no evidence to suggest that devil's claw helps or hinders arthritis. However, it may have some pain-relieving properties, so if you decide to try it, do so for several months and then reassess whether it is helpful.

DHEA

DHEA, or *dehydroepiandosterone,* is a steroid hormone that is made by the body in larger quantities than any other hormone. It is touted as a cure-all for numerous conditions, from arthritis to "aging" and everything in between.

How it's said to work: DHEA may increase the body's supply of *androgens* (male hormones), which help improve immune function. It also may have some mild anti-inflammatory properties.

Proof: The evidence for DHEA is conflicting. In studies with mice and rats, DHEA helped to reverse the decline in immune function that occurs with aging (which is why DHEA supplements have been popularized as "reversers" of the aging process). But rodents don't make any DHEA at all, so to them, any treatment with DHEA is like getting a new drug. But DHEA is very abundant in humans, on the other hand, so it should come as no surprise that the few human studies conducted have had mixed results at best. When it comes to human DHEA studies that look at arthritis in particular, the data are even sketchier. There is some evidence that women with lupus who took DHEA showed some improvement in joint achiness and fatigue, which allowed some patients to reduce their dosage of prednisone. So DHEA does show promise for lupus.

Safety issues: DHEA, a precursor to the male sex hormone *testosterone,* is thought by some researchers to have the potential to increase the incidence of prostate cancer. It also may increase the risk for endometrial cancer in women. And there is the possibility of liver damage if you are taking DHEA *and* azathioprine or methotrexate.

The bottom line: Unless you have lupus, there doesn't seem to be any evidence for or against taking DHEA for osteoarthritis or rheumatoid arthritis. If you decide to try it, do so for several months and then reassess whether it is helpful. Also, talk with your doctor. Over-the-counter DHEA preparations can vary widely in their purity, and your physician might know where to get pure sources of the compound. Most people start out with about 200 milligrams a day, but some doctors start people out on lower doses.

DMSO

DMSO, or *dimethyl sulfoxide,* is a by-product of paint thinner and antifreeze. It is commonly used in veterinary medicine for joint and tendon problems (especially in horses) and is either applied topically, right on top of the joint, or taken orally.

How it's said to work: DMSO is said to have anti-inflammatory properties, but this has never been proven.

Proof: Because of veterinary applications, DSMO has been touted as a treatment for human arthritis. In fact, it is commonly used to treat arthritis in Russia and other countries. Human studies on DMSO in the United States are few and far between and have not shown any consistent benefit.

Safety issues: In the 1960s, studies showed that using very high doses of DMSO in animals caused vision problems. No such effects have been observed in humans, but until well-designed clinical trials are conducted, the risk is hard to evaluate.

The bottom line: There is no evidence to suggest that DMSO helps or hinders arthritis, so if you decide to try it, do so for several months and then reassess whether it is helpful. But never take industrial-grade DMSO, as it may contain impurities and is probably unsafe. Talk with your doctor about finding a medical-quality preparation (also see "Resources" in the back of the book). Note that DMSO can make your breath smell like garlic, and it can cause skin irritation if applied topically.

Evening primrose oil

Evening primrose oil, along with borage and black currant seed oil, is high in a type of fatty acid called *gamma linolenic acid,* or GLA.

How it's said to work: GLA is an omega-6 fatty acid. We talked in Chapter 3 about omega-6 fatty acids and their contribution to the production of inflammatory prostaglandins. However, GLA is an exception to that rule. Some of this fatty acid can follow a different pathway and produce *anti*-inflammatory prostaglandins.

Proof: Research has been conducted with all three oils (primrose, black currant seed, and borage) on people with rheumatoid arthritis, using doses ranging from 0.5–2.8 grams of GLA a day. And while the studies have been small, the results look promising. In one 6-month study of 37 patients with rheumatoid arthritis, those who took borage seed oil had a 30–45 percent improvement in joint symptoms, 15 percent less pain, and 33 percent less morning stiffness compared to those taking a placebo. In another study, people taking evening primrose oil reported a decrease in their NSAID dosage after 12 months.

Safety issues: As with all nutrition supplements, these oils are not well regulated by the Food and Drug Administration. Therefore, you can never be sure that the label accurately reflects the contents of the bottle. Note, too, that the oils can thin the blood, so you must be cautious if you are taking blood thinners such as NSAIDs, Coumadin (warfarin), or herbs like *Ginkgo biloba.*

The bottom line: There is evidence that taking a supplement that contains GLA is helpful for people with rheumatoid arthritis. If you decide to take one of them, do so for several months and then reassess whether it is helping you. You need to take 1–2 grams of GLA daily to reach the levels that have appeared helpful in studies. That could amount to 10 capsules of borage oil daily and even more capsules of evening primrose oil. Both borage and evening primrose oil contain only *some* GLA. Look on the label to see how much GLA is present in the preparation. Ask a pharmacist if you can't figure it out. Bear in mind that all of that oil adds up to about 90 calories daily.

MSM

MSM, or *methyl sulfonyl methane,* occurs naturally in small amounts in most fresh foods, including fruits, vegetables, meat, fish, poultry, eggs, and whole milk. It is also a by-product of the breakdown of DMSO. In fact, people are now saying that it is the beneficial constituent of DMSO.

How it's said to work: Like DMSO, MSM is purported to be an anti-inflammatory agent for people with all types of arthritis.

Proof: While there have been several animal studies (research on mice has shown that MSM eases rheumatoid symptoms) and human studies without control groups, there have been no *well-controlled* human studies.

Safety issues: Because rigorous research is so scant, it can't be said with any certainty whether MSM is safe or unsafe.

The bottom line: There is no evidence to support either taking it or not taking it. Because MSM is made from DMSO, anyone considering it should make sure that the source is pure.

SAMe (pronounced *Sammy*)

SAMe, or *S-adenosylmethionine,* is produced in all humans to help perform some forty functions in the body—everything from bone preservation to proper DNA replication. Scientists in Italy first isolated SAMe in 1972. Later, while testing it in humans with depression, researchers happened to discover that subjects who had osteoarthritis were able to walk with more ease.

How it's said to work: SAMe appears to have analgesic and anti-inflammatory properties in people with osteoarthritis. People have been using it in Europe for years, but it didn't become available in the United States until 1999.

Proof: A number of animal and human studies (albeit many of them not rigorously controlled) have suggested that SAMe rebuilds eroded cartilage lining the joints by stimulating the production of the cartilage material proteoglycans. In one German trial, when researchers administered SAMe for 3 months to patients with osteoarthritis of the hands, they found significant improvement.

Safety issues: While SAMe can cause nausea or other stomach upset in large doses, it otherwise appears to be quite safe, at least over the short term. In fact, it appears to have fewer side effects than pain relievers such as ibuprofen.

The bottom line: There is evidence that SAMe may help arthritis symptoms. If you decide to take it, do so for several months and then reassess whether it is helping you. Typical doses of SAMe range from 200–400 milligrams several times per day, for a total of up to 1,600 milligrams. Look for a supplement that lists 1,4-butanedisulfate as an ingredient. That's what's used in the patented formulation of SAMe in Europe. In addition, the supplement should be enterically coated. That ensures that it will remain intact in the stomach and not dissolve until it reaches the small intestine, the organ from which it can move to the bloodstream. To improve absorption even more, some researchers recommend taking it on an empty stomach.

Stinging nettles

Nettles are wild plants whose leaves contain tiny stingers. If you brush up against them, they will cause painful stinging that usually goes away within an hour or so. People who use nettles medicinally usually boil and eat them (cooking removes the stinging quality) or take them as purified extract in capsule form. However, some people actually sting themselves with the nettles.

How it's said to work: Stinging nettles contain antioxidants, which have the potential to be helpful in the treatment of arthritis. People with arthritis who sting themselves believe that chemicals released in the "sting" will help reduce joint pain and swelling; the stinging is thought to cause an anti-inflammatory reaction.

Proof: A single controlled trial in Germany had intriguing results. Scientists gave a group of people with osteoarthritis either a typical dose of NSAIDs or a *low* dose of NSAIDs plus (boiled) nettles to eat. Pain and stiffness went down by about 70 percent in both groups, implying that stinging nettles may allow patients to reduce their NSAID dosages without exacerbating their arthritis symptoms.

Safety issues: Allergic reactions have been known to occur when stinging nettles were eaten, as is the case with most any food. Moreover, stinging yourself with nettles is painful. That pain may mask the pain of arthritis, but it probably does not actually alleviate arthritis symptoms.

The bottom line: Eating stinging nettles as food is basically just like eating any other green leafy vegetable and is perfectly healthful. It may even have some protective benefits for people with arthritis. However, we do advise against stinging yourself with nettles, as there seems to be no benefit.

THINGS YOU APPLY (OR WEAR)

Capsaicin ointment

Capsaicin is the compound that gives red peppers their heat.

How it's said to work: It is believed that capsaicin triggers the release of *endorphins,* chemicals in the body that can help provide pain relief.

Proof: One well-controlled study published in 1992 showed that capsaicin cream was beneficial to patients with osteoarthritis of the hands, reducing pain and redness. But it did not seem to help patients with rheumatoid arthritis. Even so, capsaicin cream is recommended by the American College of Rheumatology for the treatment of both osteoarthritis and rheumatoid arthritis. Doctors have used this topical cream for a number of years to treat their arthritis patients.

Safety issues: Don't *consume* excessive amounts of red peppers, that is, don't eat more peppers than you normally would with a spicy meal; it could cause indigestion. Instead, use topical capsaicin, sold over the counter or prescribed by your doctor.

The bottom line: Over-the-counter creams should contain 0.025–0.075 percent capsaicin in the ointment. Your doctor can prescribe a more potent preparation, if necessary. Apply it (after having washed your hands) directly to the painful area—but *not* to areas where there are open sores or a rash. Also, test it first on a very small spot to see if it *causes* a rash; although most people tolerate it well, some do not. Wash your hands thoroughly after you have applied the cream. You don't want to get the ointment in your eyes or other sensitive areas.

Copper bracelets

Copper bracelets have been touted as a treatment for rheumatoid arthritis for years, and many quacks have made lots of money off them. They continue to be promoted over the Internet.

How it's said to work: Copper is an essential nutrient that is necessary for the correct workings of bone. It has also been verified that dietary copper can help in the anti-inflammatory process. However, copper deficiencies are very rare—we get plenty of that mineral in our diets. Moreover, copper bracelets probably don't allow any copper to migrate through the skin for assimilation by the body, as is thought by some to occur.

Proof: There is ample proof that copper bracelets do not help people with arthritis.

Safety issues: Copper bracelets are perfectly safe.

The bottom line: Don't bother, unless you want some new jewelry.

Thera-Gesic®, Miracle Ice®, Bengay®, oil of wintergreen, and other heating ointments

All of these preparations contain *salicylic acid,* an ingredient related to aspirin.

How it's said to work: These ointments irritate the skin slightly, causing increased blood flow. That creates warmth on the skin, which soothes pain and inflammation.

Proof: All of these ointments are best used for symptoms in and around the joints. They have been recommended by rheumatologists for years because they do indeed seem to offer temporary relief from arthritis pain, although they do not prevent the damage done by arthritis.

Safety issues: Since these ointments can cause local irritation, they should not be used on rashes or broken skin.

The bottom line: Most of these over-the-counter preparations are safe and can be helpful. Just follow the manufacturers' directions, and stick with the more mainstream products.

THINGS YOU DO (OR HAVE DONE *TO* YOU)

Acupuncture

As we said in the section on Chinese herbs, according to Chinese medicine, illness occurs when a person is out of balance with nature and its two opposing forces: yin (which is feminine) and yang (which represents masculine, "forceful" qualities). Acupuncture is said to restore balance with the insertion of fine needles at particular points on meridians—fourteen pathways mapped on the body through which flows one's life force, or Qi.

How it's said to work: A panel of twelve scientists convened in 1998 by the

National Institutes of Health said that some research suggests that inserting needles into the skin (sometimes while also applying heat or electric stimulation) stimulates the release of endorphins and other opiates—natural pain relievers produced by the body. Acupuncture may also change the pattern of blood flow through the body. In one study using a sophisticated technique for measuring blood flow, a region of the brain called the *thalamus* "lit up" in people with pain who had received acupuncture treatment. Prior to acupuncture, blood flow in the thalamus was not what it should have been.

Proof: There are actually more than two hundred studies suggesting that acupuncture helps relieve various kinds of pain. One credible study, involving patients with rheumatoid arthritis, showed significant reductions in pain. Some less convincing evidence points to acupuncture as a possible treatment for osteoarthritis. Unfortunately, much of the research does not separate the results of acupuncture from any possible placebo effect. Consider that acupuncturists often spend more time with their patients than do physicians—45 minutes to an hour—and carry out their work in a soothing atmosphere unlike the doctor's office.

Safety issues: In rare instances, needles inserted as deep as an inch have made patients vulnerable to nerve and tissue damage. Also, careless handling of needles has resulted in outbreaks of hepatitis B. (The acupuncturist should use disposable needles.)

The bottom line: There is evidence that acupuncture can relieve the pain of arthritis. It has been reported that more than 1 million Americans currently use acupuncture and that a large percentage of them have painful musculoskeletal problems such as those associated with arthritis and lower back pain. But be aware that, while many states license or otherwise regulate the titles awarded to nonphysician acupuncturists, standards vary considerably. The best bet is to find out at which school the acupuncurist was trained. Then contact the American Academy of Medical Acupuncture to see if the school has been accredited (see "Resources" for more information).

Note: Most insurance companies don't cover acupuncture sessions, which typically run $40–$70, and most acupuncturists recommend at least a few sessions to give the procedure a chance to take effect.

Ayurveda

Ayurvedic medicine is an ancient practice that originated in India more than 5,000 years ago.

How it's said to work: Ayurvedic practitioners assess your constitution by looking at five life forces—earth, water, fire, air, and ether (your more spiritual side)—and then counsel you accordingly. One of the key elements of Ayurveda is working with diet to influence your digestive system so that you eliminate toxins that build up in your body. Purification diets may be prescribed for arthritis patients to remove harmful toxins and restore balance and harmony. This may all sound far-fetched, but most of Ayurvedic medicine is simply counseling on good lifestyle habits regarding diet, physical activity, and meditation.

Proof: There is very little Western scientific evidence that Ayurvedic medicine works.

Safety issues: Since Ayurvedic medicine is a mostly noninvasive practice that encourages healthful lifestyles, it is generally considered safe. However, consult your physician about any herbs or other remedies that your Ayurvedic doctor recommends. Herbs should be used with caution, as they may interfere with your medical condition or with other medications that you may be taking.

The bottom line: At the present time, there is little scientific evidence either for or against Ayurveda. But large populations of the world do use Ayurveda as a major source of medical care. Our culture has only just begun to understand this ancient type of medicine. If you decide to try Ayruveda, find a licensed practitioner (see "Resources" for more information). If after several months you see no improvement, reassess whether you are benefiting from the therapy.

Bee stings

Some people have reported reduced arthritis pain after stinging themselves with bees.

How it's said to work: Bee venom is said by some to have anti-inflammatory properties.

Proof: Research has shown that bee venom has some strong anti-

244 STRONG WOMEN AND MEN BEAT ARTHRITIS

inflammatory properties in animals. However, there are no clinical trials showing a benefit in humans.

Safety issues: Bee stings can cause fatal allergic reactions in some people, and the reactions can occur seemingly out of the blue, even after someone has been taking bee stings for a while.

The bottom line: We strongly advise against bee-sting therapy. The potential for an allergic reaction presents too great a risk, and there is little to no proven benefit.

Chiropractic

Chiropractors are the third largest body of health-care professionals in the United States, educated in any of seventeen chiropractic medical colleges. Chiropractors believe that many diseases, including musculoskeletal conditions such as arthritis, result from malalignment of the spine.

How it's said to work: The spinal manipulation practiced by chiropractors is believed to relieve arthritis pain by improving the alignment of joints.

Proof: While there is a fair amount of evidence indicating that chiropractic treatment can be effective for treating back pain, evidence for its effect on arthritis is lacking.

Safety issues: It is best to consult your medical doctor before going to a chiropractor. That's because it is important to properly diagnose the *cause* of your pain, and a regular physician is best trained to do that. Also, make sure that if you do go to a chiropractor that you choose someone who is licensed by your state and has worked with patients who have arthritis. You need to be careful because some joint manipulation can actually harm an inflamed joint. If a chiropractor claims that he or she can cure you, be wary. Arthritis cannot be "cured" per se. Be cautious, too, if the chiropractor tries to sell you products along with practicing joint manipulation. Some chiropractors augment their salaries by selling potions, herbs, and vitamin preparations.

The bottom line: The results of chiropractic medicine are comparable to those of physical therapy or other standard care for back pain. It also may be helpful for people with osteoarthritis but probably does little to ease rheumatoid arthritis pain. If you see a chiropractor, reassess after several months to see if the treatment is helping.

Tai Chi

Practiced by the Chinese for centuries, Tai Chi is a series of slow movements, or forms, that flow one into the other.

How it's said to work: Tai Chi gently exercises all the joints, muscles, and tendons in the body. It focuses on breathing and mental concentration during the performance of various movements. The relaxation brought on by the breathing and concentration allows the life force, or "Qi" (as described earlier), to flow unimpeded throughout the body. These techniques help to integrate the mind and body and allow the achievement of total harmony of the inner and outer self. Improved strength, aerobic fitness, and flexibility come with practicing Tai Chi, complementing the strength-training and aerobic activities we recommend in Chapter 5.

Proof: There has been one randomized controlled trial of Tai Chi in older adults with osteoarthritis. Practicing Tai Chi twice a week for 12 weeks resulted in small but important improvements in self-confidence, mood, and quality of life. There have also been numerous studies on Tai Chi and older individuals, with results ranging from improved balance to decreased blood pressure. In a smaller study, Tai Chi improved strength in the quadriceps and hamstring muscles by 15–20 percent.

Safety issues: Tai Chi is very safe. In fact, it's often recommended for people who are unable or unwilling to do other kinds of exercise. The key to following a Tai Chi program is to make sure that you start out slowly and that the movements don't cause any more pain than you usually experience. As you get stronger and more flexible, you will be able to do more aggressive moves.

The bottom line: There is evidence that Tai Chi is beneficial for people with arthritis, and we encourage you to try it. Your local "Y," health club, or senior citizens center probably offers a Tai Chi class. Your state Arthritis Foundation can also recommend a qualified teacher. But before you sign on, make sure that the other participants in the class are in similar physical shape and health so that the level is consistent with your needs. Also, get your doctor's approval. Tai Chi can be physically demanding. Your primary care physician will know whether you're taking medications that could interfere with balance or create a condition that could make a series of Tai Chi movements unadvisable. You can also buy a Tai Chi video if you want to do the exercises at home (see "Resources" for suggestions).

Yoga

The practice of yoga, which originated in India more than 2,000 years ago, involves a variety of static postures, or *asanas,* which include backward and forward bends as well as twisted positions. These movements, while meant to increase the mind's capacity for concentration and meditation, also emphasize physical conditioning.

How it's said to work: By increasing flexibility, range of motion, and bone and muscle strength, yoga may be able to reduce arthritis pain. The postures are also said to align bones and muscles.

Proof: While some yoga books have included specific recommendations for the treatment of arthritis, little objective evidence exists. Only two small controlled trials have been reported. In one, people with osteoarthritis of the hands who practiced yoga for 10 weeks showed significantly greater improvement in pain and joint tenderness as well as range of motion compared to a group that did not do yoga. In the other study, yoga was better than a standard wrist splint at reducing pain and improving grip strength in the hands.

Safety issues: The key is to find yoga positions that provide force for muscle strengthening and flexibility but are not detrimental to the joint. Overzealous students can hurt themselves by trying to master a difficult pose too quickly.

The bottom line: There is evidence that yoga is beneficial for people with arthritis, and we encourage you to try it. As with Tai Chi, you can often locate a yoga class at your local "Y" or fitness center, but finding the right instructor is a bit of a hit-or-miss proposition. There is no standardized certification program for yoga teachers. Your best bet is to look for someone with extended teaching experience and an interest in working with those with special needs, such as people with arthritis. Note that *Iyengar* yoga, a type of *hatha* yoga (which is what most Americans envision when they think of yoga), works especially well for people with physical limitations because it allows for the use of props like blocks, belts, and other supports to help achieve poses more easily and with less risk of injury (see "Resources").

No matter what complementary therapy you may try, proceed cautiously. And think of it as a complementary treatment—not a substitute for sound

Sham therapies

Unfortunately, desperation for relief from a condition such as arthritis leads to the proliferation of treatments for which there is no proof of benefit other than to the pocketbooks of those advocating the particular therapy. A number of these so-called therapies persist despite the lack of help they have provided, serving only to steer people away from treatments that could really help—and using up their money in the bargain. Following is a list of some these useless therapies.

- Coenzyme Q10
- Gin-soaked raisins
- Low-energy laser therapy
- Magnets
- Copper bracelets

There are probably many more that we haven't mentioned here!

medical management of your condition. If a therapy seems to help you, continue with it. If it doesn't, stop.

Liz tried bee stings for a while and says that although "there were times that it *felt* like it helped, in the long run I don't think it did." So she stopped. On the other hand, Earl, the fireman who had his hip replaced, says that he can feel a difference with 1,500 milligrams a day of glucosamine and "will continue to take it." Both consulted with their physicians in making their decisions. Partnering with your own physician, you'll be able to make the right decisions for yourself.

The Beat Arthritis Workbook

———— ■ ————

While Sister Mary Patrice was enrolled in the Tufts study, Kristin encouraged her (as well as all the other participants) to keep written records of how the exercise program was going. Charting the changes in strength and energy, Kristin felt, would motivate people to stay with the plan—even if they didn't always accomplish what they would have liked in a given period of time. It worked.

"I thought it was very helpful to see my progress on paper," Sister Mary Patrice relates. 'You can see what works, what doesn't. Also, you could gauge how things were going. Two weeks ago I was able to do a lift nine times. Now I'm up to twelve.' It helped even to write things down on a day that I didn't do so well because of pain," Sister Mary Patrice says. "That way, I could see what was going on."

Liz kept records, too. She was able to rattle off to us that she walked 579 miles in 1999. She knew, too, that she was up to 10- to 12-pound weights by the time she stopped strength training at home and started going to the gym. She also had records of when she tried, as she calls it, "the whole gamut of drugs—the Plaquenil, the gold shots, Feldene, prednisone, methotrexate—including when the doctor would change doses." That enabled her to figure out what was really working (in her case, it was Enbrel, finally, that made a significant difference and allowed her to get the most out of the exercise program).

This kind of record keeping really improves your chances for success. After all, we have given you a lot of information in this book about a lot of different ways to reduce your pain and get you more mobile. An easy system for tracking the changes as you go will help you to pull it all together. So, just as we would do if you were with us in one of our studies at Tufts, we're going to give you some tools for measuring your improvements.

First, we're going to have you take a few self-assessments. Then, you'll keep track of them over the first 16 weeks of the program—and periodically after that, as you see fit. You'll see—these assessments, or questionnaires, will be very helpful for you in gauging your progress.

In addition to the questionnaires, we have created logs for you to keep for exercise and nutrition to help you see specifically, from day to day and week to week, where you are in terms of your goals. Research continues to show that keeping logs is one of the single best ways to enhance compliance with an exercise and nutrition program.

The following chart summarizes, in the most basic terms, our recommendations for managing your arthritis symptoms. They include the core components of the program that you will be assessing and keeping track of.

Summary of how to manage the symptoms of your arthritis

Exercise
- Strength training
- Aerobic—weight bearing if not painful
- Stretching—a must, or you will not see optimal results and may set yourself up for injury

Note for inflammatory arthritis patients: When you have a flare-up, drop down a progression on your strength training, shorten your aerobic workouts, but continue doing your flexibility exercises.

Nutrition
- Weight loss if needed (for individuals with osteoarthritis)
- Follow the Arthritis Food Guide Pyramid (page 55)
- Take a multivitamin supplement
- Consider taking 400 IU of vitamin D and 200–800 IU of vitamin E
- Consider taking fish oil capsules if you have rheumatoid arthritis

Medication (as directed by a physician)
- Nonsteroidal anti-inflammatory drugs (NSAIDs)
- Acetaminophen
- Oral or injected steroids when needed
- DMARDs (disease-modifying anti-rheumatic drugs) for inflammatory arthritis

Complementary Therapy
While there are many different types of complementary therapies to consider, we feel there is the most promise in these:

- Glucosamine/chondroitin supplements (for osteoarthritis)
- Yoga/Tai Chi
- Acupuncture
- SAMe (for individuals with osteoarthritis)
- Heating ointments
- Borage, evening primrose, or black currant oil (for inflammatory arthritis)
- Chiropractic

Medical Care (as directed by a physician)
- Joint replacement surgery, if necessary
- Evaluation of new procedures aside from joint replacement surgery
- Physical therapy (when necessary)
- Occupational therapy (when necessary)

BEFORE YOU BEGIN THE PROGRAM

If any one of us were to work with you on an individual basis, we would start by asking you a few questions. Specifically, we would want to know the following:

- Your body mass index (BMI)
- How much pain you are in right now
- How well you function physically in your everyday life (and if your arthritis limits you)
- Your medications and medical care
- To what degree, if any, you feel depressed
- Your eating habits
- Your current level of physical activity

These are the things that we are going to help you find out right now. Answer these questionnaires—they will help you determine the exact "prescription" for your own program as well as enable you to carefully monitor your progress.

Measure your body mass index (BMI)

Your BMI, which we discussed in greater detail in Chapter 3, is a single number that takes into consideration both your height and your weight. It lets you know whether you are overweight.

To find out your BMI, first have someone measure your height without shoes and socks, preferably first thing in the morning. (That's the time of day you're tallest—the tug of gravity makes you up to a half-inch shorter by evening.) Next, weigh yourself. Finally, refer to the chart on pages 42–43 in Chapter 3 and locate your BMI. Record it on the assessment sheet on page 259.

Even if your body weight is fairly stable, it is a good idea to weigh yourself a few times a year. It can alert you to unwanted increases—the sooner you discover a change, the easier it is to correct. You also need to know about slow decreases, which can sometimes be a sign of medical problems. Most people reach a peak body weight in their fifties and sixties, then slowly lose weight in their seventies, eighties, and nineties.

Evaluate your current pain

Whenever we work with arthritis patients, we want to assess their current level of pain. If you are in a lot of pain right now, you may need to start extra slowly to make sure that you don't aggravate your symptoms. If your level of pain is unbearable, you should *definitely* discuss with your doctor the advisability of starting an exercise program. No matter what, be patient. You can at least start to *eat* better no matter what your level of pain. In fact, we have seen over and over again that exercise *and* better nutrition help to reduce pain. Use the scale below to measure your pain level.

0	2	4	6	8	10
No pain	Mild	Moderate	Severe	Unbearable

The scale goes from 0 to 10, with 0 indicating no pain at all, 2 indicating mild pain, 5 indicating moderate pain, 7 indicating severe pain, and 10 indicating extreme, unbearable pain. Remember that you can also fit anywhere in between these numbers: For instance, if you feel that you are somewhere between mild and moderate, maybe you are a 3.5. Determine the average amount of pain you have been feeling in the past week and mark accordingly along the line. You will be asked to do a follow-up every 4 weeks you are on the program. This will be described later in the chapter.

Evaluate your physical function

Understanding where you are in terms of your ability to function physically in your everyday life is important because it lets you know how well the program is working for you. Respond according to your level of physical function over the past week by filling out the brief questionnaire below, then total your score. You will do follow-up assessments on this chart as you progress in the program. This will be described later in the chapter.

Rate your physical functional ability for the six questions below as follows:

1—no limitations at all
2—some limitations
3—a lot of limitations

Score:

_____ Vigorous activities, such as running, sports (soccer, basketball, singles tennis, strenuous hiking)

_____ Moderate activities, such as housecleaning (scrubbing floors, vacuuming, moving furniture), golf, gardening, bowling, leisurely biking

_____ Climbing two or more flights of stairs

_____ Carrying and lifting groceries

_____ Walking several blocks

_____ Walking more than a mile

_____ **Total score**

Lower scores (less than 10) indicate good physical function. Moderate scores (10–13) indicate fair physical function. Higher scores (14–18) indicate poorer physical function. Even a change of as little as one point can have dramatic effects on the quality of your life.

Take stock of your medications and medical care

By answering the following questions and then answering them again later on, you'll get a sense of how well our program is working in tandem with your doctor's care and any drugs you might be taking.

1. How often do you see your primary care physician?

_____

2. If you see a rheumatologist, how often do you see him or her?

_____

3. Do you see any other types of health professionals for your arthritis, such as a physical therapist, chiropractor, or acupuncturist? If so, how often?

_____

4. What medications, if any, do you take for your arthritis? What is the daily dose?

Medication: _____ Dose: _____

Medication: _____ Dose: _____

Medication: _____ Dose: _____
Medication: _____ Dose: _____

Are you suffering from depression?

It is important to know if you are clinically depressed. If you are, it will be a large obstacle in accomplishing your exercise and nutrition goals and will set you up for frustration and possible failure unless you take steps to address it. Note that depression is sometimes masked by other symptoms, and many people don't recognize that they have a problem. The checklist below will help you determine if you should seek help for depression, say, by asking your physician to refer you to a psychiatrist, psychologist, or social worker.

If you answer yes to any of the following, contact your health-care provider for referral to a specialist. You may be depressed or at risk for depression.

_____ Yes   _____ No   Persistent sad mood
_____ Yes   _____ No   Loss of interest or pleasure in activities that were once enjoyed
_____ Yes   _____ No   Significant change in appetite or body weight
_____ Yes   _____ No   Difficulty sleeping—or oversleeping
_____ Yes   _____ No   Significant increase in irritability
_____ Yes   _____ No   Marked loss of energy
_____ Yes   _____ No   Feelings of worthlessness or burdensome guilt
_____ Yes   _____ No   Difficulty thinking or concentrating
_____ Yes   _____ No   Recurrent thoughts of death or suicide

Assess your eating habits

Evaluate your typical eating habits. This will spell out clearly where you are doing well and where your diet needs upgrading. Use the Arthritis Food Guide Pyramid on page 55, and at the end of the day recall what you ate and jot down how many servings from each category you had. In addition, look at the number of vitamin C– and beta-carotene–rich foods you ate. Pages 59 and 60 list these nutrient-rich foods, respectively. Compare your results to the recommendations listed here as well as in Chapter 4 on Nutrition.

Food Pyramid Checklist (recall all the foods you ate over the last day)
Number of servings (check out pages 56–57 if you can't remember how large a serving is):

		Daily Goal
_____	Water or other noncaffeinated drinks	8
_____	Fruits and vegetables	6 or more
_____	Whole grains	2 or more
_____	Processed grains	no more than 3
_____	Fish, legumes, and soy foods	1 or more
_____	Meats	2 or less
_____	Dairy foods (or calcium-enriched soy milk)	2 to 3
_____	Junk foods (sweets, chips, candy, etc.)	1 or less

Is this a typical day? If not, do the recall for one more day this week.

Evaluate your physical activity

Assessing your current exercise habits can help you determine the best goals for planning an effective fitness program and staying on track. We realize that many of you may not be doing any exercise right now. That's fine. Remember that our program is going to progress slowly, and by the end of 16 weeks you will be so much fitter than you might think possible at the moment. Record your answers regarding your physical activity during the previous week.

		Goal
Average number of (aerobic) sessions per week:	_____	3 sessions
Average minutes/session:	_____	20 minutes
Types of aerobic exercise:	_____	
Average number of strength-training sessions per week:	_____	3 sessions
Do I stretch after each workout or at all?	_____ Yes _____	No

Set realistic goals

Comparing where you're at right now with where you should be, write down as many details as you can about your goals (what type of exercises you will do, how many times per week you are willing to commit to exercise at the start, how many fruits and vegetables you will strive to eat each day, how many servings of fish you will eat each week, whether to make a doctor's appointment, etc.). Make sure these goals are within your reach. The idea is not to try to accomplish everything at once. That will only set you up for frustration and unnecessary feelings of failure. For instance, if you never walked for exercise before, you're not going to walk 2 miles at the end of a week.

The way to make sure your goals are appropriate is to be as specific as possible. The first week, can you eat one more vegetable per day than you usually do? Two? Will you walk for 10 minutes a day every other day? How many strength-training exercises will you start out with per session? You know yourself best! Of course, remember that your goals should change as you progress.

Exercise _____

_____

_____

Nutrition _____

_____

Doctors' appointments _____
Other _____

_____

Don't forget the triggers!

If you have not already done so, use the diary in Chapter 6 (pages 180–181) to help you identify your negative triggers—and your solutions for turning them into positives so that you will engage in the positive behaviors necessary for reaching your goals. Remember that negative triggers are those cognitive, emotional, environmental, physical, and social obstacles that keep you from exercising and/or eating well.

Negative Triggers	Positive Responses to Triggers
_____	_____
_____	_____
_____	_____
_____	_____
_____	_____

Reassessment at four-week intervals

Now that you've answered all the questionnaires, you have your baseline—the place you start from. From here on, the point is to reevaluate where you are every 4 weeks, which is exactly what we'd ask you to do if we were working with you on an individual basis. That'll show you just how far you've come and where you still want to make improvements. For instance, perhaps you're now at two vegetables a day and want to try to increase it to three. Or maybe you're doing only some of the components of the strength-training sessions each week and need a plan for expanding to full sessions. Or maybe it's time to discuss something about your medications with your doctor.

The 15-Minute Monthly Self-Assessment Checklist on the following pages makes it easy to do. In just 15 minutes every 4 weeks, you can see at a glance exactly where you were and where you're at currently. You'll be surprised at how motivating the improvement in your health will be.

We encourage you to do the self-assessment exactly every 4 weeks. For example, if you start on May 3, reassess on May 31, then June 28, and so on.

IT DOESN'T HAVE TO FEEL OVERWHELMING

As you read this book, we hope you have decided to change your diet, to consider taking nutritional supplements, to begin several different kinds of physical exercise. Some people meet such challenges very easily. But there are a lot of different components to this, and many of us find it difficult to face numerous tasks all at once. We feel overwhelmed; we procrastinate.

It doesn't have to be that way. In our experience—and there's research to back us up—there are two simple secrets to success: make your plans specific and keep logs.

Reevaluate your needs when life gets complicated

Sophie was diagnosed with osteoarthritis of the hip and was 2 months into the program when her husband had a stroke. This time in her life was tremendously stressful, both emotionally and physically. Sophie had progressed so much over the 2 months, but her life had been turned upside down, and now her husband demanded 100 percent of her attention. She completely stopped the program. But Kristin then worked with her to figure out a very targeted, small program that she could follow with ease.

As the demands on her time were much greater, Sophie had to re-work her immediate goals—and the steps to achieve them—in order to fit the program back into her life. Kristin recommended that she cut back on her strengthening workout and do only the key exercises, which took her just 15 minutes instead of 40. Later in the day she would take another breather and do 5–10 minutes of stretching. On days she did not strength-train, she tried to take a 10-minute walk outside as a breather for herself.

It was only a couple of weeks before Sophie realized she could withstand the stress better and be more helpful to her husband and others if she took some time for herself. Emotionally and physically she felt so much more capable, and she had more energy to care for her husband.

Even at times when we feel there is no way to find the time to take care of ourselves, in the long run it proves to serve not just us better but also those around us. Even if you stick with just one small component of the program, it will be so much easier to get back on track when your life calms down.

Make your plans specific

Don't just *decide* you're going to do something; write it out on paper. The more specific you make your plans by writing them down, the easier it will be to follow through. Start by completing the questionnaires on pages 251–257.

THE *STRONG WOMEN* AND MEN *BEAT ARTHRITIS* 15-MINUTE MONTHLY SELF-ASSESSMENT CHECKLIST

Body Mass Index (BMI)

Starting BMI _____   Goal BMI _____

Week 4 _____   Week 8 _____

Week 12 _____   Week 16 _____

Pain assessment

Make note of your pain score (from the 0–10 point scale on page 252). Record your pain score on the graph below at the start of the program and then every 4 weeks thereafter.

| | Start | Week 4 | Week 8 | Week 12 | Week 16 |

0 = no pain; 5 = moderate; 10 = unbearable

Then set aside another 30 minutes to make plans. Sit down with this book, your calendar, and a pad and pencil, and go back over the forms you filled out.

What changes are you going to make in your diet? Compose a shopping list (see page 261). Have you decided to try flaxseed oil? If so, make sure your supermarket has it, or find one that does. Figure out what dishes you are going to use it in (a dip for fresh vegetables?), and decide when you are going to make it.

What about exercise? Do you need to buy equipment? Weights? Sneakers? Make a list, and order by mail. Or check the Yellow Pages and put a shopping appointment on your calendar. It may sound too simple to bother with, but

PHYSICAL FUNCTIONAL ASSESSMENT

Using the physical function assessment from page 252–253, record your
score on the graph below when you start the program and then every
4 weeks thereafter. Remember that lower scores indicate better function.

18					
15					
12					
9					
6					
	Start	Week 4	Week 8	Week 12	Week 16

NOTE YOUR ACCOMPLISHMENTS

Week 4:
Medications/medical care _____
Nutrition _____
Exercise _____
Other (including mood) _____

Week 8:
Medications/medical care _____
Nutrition _____
Exercise _____
Other (including mood) _____

Week 12:
Medications/medical care _____
Nutrition _____
Exercise _____
Other (including mood) _____

Week 16:
Medications/medical care _____
Nutrition _____
Exercise _____
Other (including mood) _____

THE BEAT ARTHRITIS SHOPPING LIST

DAIRY
- ☐ low-fat/non-fat milk
- ☐ low-fat/non-fat yogurt
- ☐ cheeses
- ☐ frozen yogurt

SOY PRODUCTS, BEANS, NUTS, AND SEEDS
- ☐ soy milk (with calcium added)
- ☐ soybeans, soy nuts
- ☐ edamame
- ☐ tofu made with calcium sulfate
- ☐ beans, dry or canned (kidney, black, navy, chickpeas, pintos, lentils, butter beans, black-eyed peas, navy, field peas, split peas)
- ☐ nuts/seeds (almonds, walnuts, butternuts, pecans, flaxseeds)

GRAINS
- ☐ whole-grain breads
- ☐ whole-grain pasta
- ☐ brown rice
- ☐ fortified whole-grain cereals
- ☐ wheat germ
- ☐ Rolled oats (oatmeal)

VEGETABLES
- ☐ spinach
- ☐ Swiss chard
- ☐ kale
- ☐ collard greens
- ☐ bok choy
- ☐ mixed lettuce greens
- ☐ romaine
- ☐ red/green leaf
- ☐ watercress
- ☐ arugula
- ☐ endive
- ☐ escarole
- ☐ chicory
- ☐ radicchio
- ☐ green beans
- ☐ broccoli
- ☐ cauliflower
- ☐ squash (zucchini and yellow)
- ☐ carrots
- ☐ peas (snap peas and sugar peas)
- ☐ cabbage
- ☐ peppers (red, orange, yellow, and green)
- ☐ tomatoes
- ☐ winter squash (butternut, acorn, spaghetti)
- ☐ sweet potatoes
- ☐ white potatoes
- ☐ vegetable juice
- ☐ frozen vegetables

FRUITS/JUICES
- ☐ calcium-fortified juice
- ☐ orange juice
- ☐ oranges
- ☐ grapefruits
- ☐ tangerines
- ☐ mangoes
- ☐ kiwis
- ☐ apples
- ☐ pears
- ☐ peaches
- ☐ plums
- ☐ bananas
- ☐ melons (watermelon, cantaloupe, honeydew)
- ☐ pineapples
- ☐ strawberries
- ☐ blueberries

OILS/FATS
- ☐ canola oil
- ☐ flaxseed oil
- ☐ olive oil
- ☐ almond butter

FISH
- ☐ fresh salmon
- ☐ mackerel
- ☐ halibut
- ☐ herring
- ☐ tuna
- ☐ trout
- ☐ swordfish
- ☐ bluefish
- ☐ canned fish (salmon, tuna, sardines)

if you don't choose a day to purchase what you need, that day might never come.

Figure out, too, which days and what times you plan to exercise, and add those appointments to your calendar as well.

Take your exercise and nutrition goals—*and* the negative and positive trigger list—and post it where you will see it every day, like the refrigerator.

You are obviously not going to buy all this food, but the list serves as a reminder of the number of food choices out there—a lot that you probably have not tried. Experiment to bring not only good nutrition but also variety to your diet.

Buy enough fresh vegetables to last only a few days, as they will lose many of their nutrients if you keep them around longer. Try to buy them twice a week. Keep your freezer stocked with frozen vegetables so that when fresh are not available, you have the next best thing, and you will not run shy on your six–plus a day. Frozen fruits, such as frozen berries to put on top of yogurt or even ice cream, can supplement your fresh-fruit selections. Canned fruits in their own juices are a good option, too.

Keep Logs

The self-assessments we've shown you so far are to be taken every 4 weeks. But it's also important to fill out exercise and nutrition logs on a *daily* basis. Don't worry—it takes, literally, only a minute or two a day. But studies have shown over and over again that spending that minute a day to record what you've done as part of the program is the single most effective method for assuring success. Make photocopies of the logs on pages 264–266, and put them in a folder or on the fridge.

Nutrition logs

Many of our research volunteers like to tape their food logs to the fridge. Use them not only for foods you eat at home but also for everything you eat while out of the house, whether at a restaurant or on the run. You might want to start by filling out the log for a week *before* you start the program to get a better sense of where you need to tweak your eating habits. Use the Arthritis Food Guide Pyramid (page 55) as your guide as you fill out the food log. Once eating better becomes second nature, you won't need to fill out the logs as often.

Exercise logs

The exercise program in this book involves three separate components: strength training, aerobics, and flexibility movements. Within the strength-training component alone, there are ten or more different exercises once you have been in the program for 16 weeks. That's a lot to keep track of, so it's a good idea to write down from day to day what you've accomplished. Of course, you'll make progress as you go along and therefore will need to adjust the amount of weight you lift as well as the length and intensity of your aerobic workouts. Written records will make doing that so much more efficient. And there's a bonus in it: It will be so satisfying to look back at your earlier logs a few months down the line and see just how far you've come!

For those of you who follow a different program because of the type of arthritis you have or the severity of the disease, we have included a blank exercise log for you to use (page 266). Simply fill in the exercises that you do.

IF YOU NEED INDIVIDUAL HELP

The "Resources" section of this book contains a list of books and organizations that can provide extra support or information. But sometimes working one-on-one with a health professional other than your primary care physician or rheumatologist can also prove valuable. And it doesn't necessarily have to cost a fortune. Your health insurance may cover a number of visits, especially if your physician writes a letter documenting how the extra professional care will help you and save the insurance company health-care dollars in the long run.

There are five kinds of specialists you might want to consider:

Registered dietitian

A registered dietitian will work with you to help you adjust your eating habits in accordance with your own food likes and dislikes. She or he will also show you how to incorporate healthful choices into your food plan with the least amount of fuss both at the supermarket and in the kitchen, and will give solid advice for choosing healthfully when eating out. Make sure the person you see is a registered dietitian, with the letters R.D. after her or his name. In most states, just about anyone can hang out a shingle bearing the

STRONG WOMEN AND MEN *BEAT ARTHRITIS*
Weekly Food Log

	GOAL	SUN	MON	TUES	WED	THU	FRI	SAT
Fluids Water, juice, noncaf-feinated beverages	8 glasses/ day							
Fruits and vegetables	At least 6/day							
Grains At least half from whole grains	4–9/day							
	Whole grains							
	Refined grains							
Fish, legumes, and soy foods	At least 1/day							
Meats	≤ 2/day							
Dairy foods (or soy products fortified with calcium)	2–3/day							
Junk foods	≤ 1/day							

Notes:

STRONG WOMEN AND MEN BEAT ARTHRITIS Weekly Exercise Log								
EXERCISE	GOAL *(fill in)*	SUN	MON	TUES	WED	THU	FRI	SAT
Aerobic activity (minutes)	3 times/week							
Strength training (12 reps × 2 sets)	3 times/week	Fill in pounds or progression for each session						
Modified squat								
Step-up								
Ankle flexion								
Modified push-up								
*Back extension								
*Modified boat pose								
Knee extension								
Knee flexion								
Reverse fly								
Lateral shoulder raises								
Stretches (2 × 30 seconds each) Lunge Hamstring Crossover Quadriceps Shoulder stretch	After each workout							

*Note: For back extension and modified boat pose, perform only 5 repetitions. You will progress by increasing the time from 10 seconds per repetition to 20 seconds per repetition (as described in Chapter 5, pages 108–111).

Weekly Exercise Log

Exercise	Goal *(fill in)*	Sun	Mon	Tues	Wed	Thu	Fri	Sat
Aerobic activity (minutes)	3 times/ week							
Strength training (12 reps × 2 sets)	3 times/ week	Fill in pounds or progression for each session						
Stretches (2 × 30 seconds each) Lunge Hamstring Crossover Quadriceps Shoulder stretch	After each workout							

title "nutritionist." But an R.D. has been through rigorous training and has passed a difficult examination administered by the American Dietetic Association. To find an R.D. in your area, contact the American Dietetic Association at (800) 366-1655 or www.eatright.org.

Personal trainer

Hiring a personal trainer might seem extravagant, but you might be able to get a lot of valuable mileage out of just a couple of sessions, keeping costs down. A personal trainer can help you make sure you're isolating the right muscles during each of your strength-training exercises and can also be called in for another session should you want to change your routine later on. Also, some personal trainers are specially skilled in helping people whose physical limitations may necessitate various exercise adaptations. Working with a personal trainer, even if only briefly, can be a great motivator.

You can always get a referral to a personal trainer from a local health club. Senior citizen centers sometimes recommend personal trainers as well. Try to make sure the trainer you choose has worked with people who have arthritis. Also, verify that he or she has been certified by at least one of the follow organizations: the American College of Sports Medicine, the National Strength and Conditioning Association, the National Academy of Sports Medicine, the American Council on Exercise, the Aerobics and Fitness Association of America, or the International Association of Fitness Professionals (IDEA).

Physical therapist

Physical therapists are highly trained professionals who work with individuals just like you. They are specially trained to help you work through specific joint problems. If you have a particular problem that goes beyond the scope of this book, talk to your doctor about getting a referral to one. (See "Resources" for more information.)

Occupational therapist

Occupational therapists (OTs) are skilled, licensed health professionals who assist people who, for one reason or another, are unable to function independently. If, for instance, someone with arthritis is having difficulty with activities of daily living, such as dressing, eating, cooking, or bathing, an occupational therapist can help. He or she will be able to recommend various assistance devices and also will know how to perform joint splinting to relieve pain. OTs usually work on the joints of the arms and feet, but a good one will treat the whole body. Talk to your doctor or see "Resources" to locate a licensed OT.

Psychotherapist

If you have any of the symptoms listed under the "Depression" discussion on page 254, we urge you to talk to a mental health professional. There is no stigma attached. Taking care of body *and* mind are both part of good health care. Therapy doesn't have to last forever. A few sessions with a trained therapist can help you sort out and deal with a lot of negative feelings. Good referral sources include your doctor and the psychology or psychiatry department at a local teaching hospital.

You are about to embark on a health program that is literally going to change your life. But you're not just going to be in less pain from arthritis. You're going to end up feeling stronger and more able to tackle the world than you have in years. You're going to sleep better and therefore feel more rested. You're going to eat better, which not only will help you cope with arthritis but also will assist you in losing excess weight, if necessary, and go a long way toward staving off chronic, debilitating conditions such as heart disease and diabetes. You're also going to feel younger and more in charge of your life.

Some of the changes will come quickly. Within 2 weeks, you'll start to feel stronger. Some will come more slowly, but that's okay. If you keep working at it, you'll start to see the differences—especially when you look back as you track your progress and see the "distance" you've covered!

It's a lifestyle commitment worth making. As Liz says, "You don't just have to live with the cards you're dealt. There's a lot you can do to change the hand."

Glossary

— ◆ —

Alpha-linolenic acid: an unsaturated fatty acid that is an essential nutrient in our diet and is found in large quantities in flaxseed oil (and in smaller amounts in fish, tofu, nuts, seeds, and green leafy vegetables). It is an omega-3 fatty acid.

Antioxidant: a nutrient or chemical that "absorbs" damage caused by free radicals, thereby protecting body tissues.

Arthritis: inflammation in a joint.

Atrophy: loss of mass of muscle, tendon, or other body structure.

Autoimmune disease: any of several diseases caused by the body's own immune system.

Beta-carotene: a form of vitamin A found primarily in fruits and vegetables.

Body mass index: a measure of weight for height. The most common way to determine BMI is to divide weight (in kilograms) by height squared (in meters). To see your BMI, refer to pages 42–43.

Cachexia: loss of muscle mass.

Cartilage: a layer of connective tissue cells covering the ends of each bone inside a joint.

Chondrocytes: cells that secrete cartilage.

Collagen: strong "ropelike" connective tissue that acts as scaffolding in bones, joints, and skin.

Cytokine: a protein molecule made by white blood cells to "communicate" between those cells.

Daily values: nutrition guidelines developed by the Food and Drug Administration for use on food labels.

Docosohexanoeic acid (DHA): a highly unsaturated fatty acid found in cold-water fish. This is an omega-3 fatty acid with anti-inflammatory properties.

Eicosapentonoeic acid (EPA): a highly unsaturated fatty acid also found in cold-water fish. It can be manufactured to some degree in the body from alpha-linolenic acid. This is an omega-3 fatty acid with anti-inflammatory properties.

Enzymes: compounds that help chemical reactions occur but are not themselves used up in the reaction.

Fatty acid: a carbon chain of varying length that is the major component of fat. There are many different types of fatty acids.

Free radicals: highly reactive by-products of metabolism that can be harmful to the body in large amounts.

Hormone: a protein molecule produced by a gland that signals the body to perform a metabolic function.

Immune system: the body system responsible for healing injuries, fighting infections, and detecting and destroying tumors before they get established.

Inflammation: pain, swelling, and redness caused by immune cells in response to injury or autoimmune disease.

Juvenile Chronic Arthritis: inflammatory arthritis in children under age 16.

Lupus: an autoimmune disease affecting joints, skin, or internal organs.

Metabolism: the sum of all the chemical reactions in the body, involving proteins, carbohydrates, fats, and DNA and RNA.

Methotrexate: a common disease-modifying anti-inflammatory drug.

Microklutz: a minor misstep that leads to joint pain because the muscles fail to tense properly and protect the joint.

Monoarticular: involving only one joint.

Muscle wasting: atrophy of muscles that is usually due to inflammation, malnutrition, and/or disease.

NSAIDs (nonsteroidal anti-inflammatory drugs): medications that reduce pain and inflammation but do not prevent the progression of arthritis.

Omega-9 fatty acid: a monounsaturated fatty acid found in high concentrations in olive, peanut, and canola oils. It has been suggested that omega-9 fatty acid may also have anti-inflammatory properties.

Omega-6 fatty acids: a family of fatty acids that is essential to human health and is contained in cottonseed, safflower, and corn oils. Excess omega-6 fatty acids result in increased inflammation. The consumption of omega-6 fatty acids has increased greatly over the last 50 years due to the increased availability of highly processed foods. Currently our diet contains large quantities of these fatty acids.

Omega-3 fatty acids: a family of fatty acids that is essential to human health and is found in large quantities in cold-water fish and flaxseed oil (and in smaller amounts in tofu, nuts, seeds, and green leafy vegetables). Omega-3 fatty acids have anti-inflammatory properties. The intake of these fatty acids in our diet has declined greatly since the mid-1800s.

Osteoarthritis: the most common type of arthritis, a degenerative disease causing inflammation inside but not outside the joints.

Pannus: an invasive layer of inflammatory cells around the joint in rheumatoid arthritis.

Pauciarticular: involving two to three joints.

Polyarticular: involving three or more joints.

Prostaglandins: fatty acid derivatives that are used as signal molecules within and between cells.

Proteoglycans: molecules of connective tissue in cartilage.

Pseudogout: arthritis caused by deposition of calcium phosphate crystals.

Rheumatoid arthritis: the most common type of inflammatory arthritis and one that usually affects many joints, including those of the hands and feet.

Rheumatologist: a physician who specializes in arthritis and related diseases.

Seronegative spondyloarthropathies: a group of inflammatory arthritises distinct from rheumatoid arthritis that usually affect the spine and large joints.

Sjögren's syndrome: an autoimmune disease that causes dry eyes and mouth.

Strength training: a mode of exercise in which the muscle works against resistance enough to increase strength.

Synovial fluid: fluid inside joints that normally lubricates them and enables nutrients to get into the cartilage.

Systemic disease: a disease that affects more than one body system.

Vitamins: nutrients that cannot be synthesized by the body and must be obtained from the diet.

Weight-bearing exercise: a mode of exercise, such as walking, in which the legs support body weight.

X-ray: a form of radiation that passes through the body and can be used to obtain images of bone and joints.

Resources

■

Following is a list of organizations, names and addresses, books, and websites that will lead you to more information on particular issues pertaining to arthritis. Please bear in mind that websites come and go. The sites listed here were accessible when we compiled this section. If any one of them is inoperative, use a reliable search engine to locate the source at its new site.

Dr. Nelson's website and books

www.strongwomen.com has a free electronic newsletter as well as other useful information regarding nutrition and exercise.

Strong Women Stay Slim. Miriam E. Nelson, Ph.D., with Sarah Wernick, Ph.D. (New York: Bantam Books, 1998).

Strong Women Stay Young. rev. ed. Miriam E. Nelson, Ph.D., with Sarah Wernick, Ph.D. (New York: Bantam Books, 2000).

Strong Women, Strong Bones. Miriam E. Nelson, Ph.D., with Sarah Wernick, Ph.D. (New York: Putnam, 2000).

Strong Women Eat Well. Miriam E. Nelson, Ph.D., with Judy Knipe (New York: Putnam, 2001).

General arthritis resources

The American Academy of Orthopaedic Surgeons has information about treatments for arthritis including surgery. You can also locate a surgeon in your area on the website.

American Academy of Orthopaedic Surgeons
6300 North River Road
Rosemont, IL 60018-4262
Ph: 847-823-7186 or 800-346-AAOS
Fax: 847-823-8125
www.aaos.org

The American College of Rheumatology lists the names of doctors who are board-certified rheumatologists.

American College of Rheumatology
1800 Century Place, Suite 250
Atlanta, GA 30345
Ph: 404-633-3777
Fax: 404-633-1870
www.rheumatology.org

The Arthritis Foundation is the leading national governing organization on arthritis. It also has an excellent website.

Arthritis Foundation
P.O. Box 7669
Atlanta, GA 30357-0669
Ph: 404-827-7100
www.arthritis.org

General nutrition resources

The Tufts University Health & Nutrition Letter, an 8-page monthly newsletter, has been called "the best available source of news and views on nutrition" by *U.S. News & World Report* and has also received accolades from *The New York Times, The Boston Globe,* the *Columbia Journalism Review,* and other publications.

Tufts University Health & Nutrition Letter
10 High Street, Suite 706
Boston, MA 02110
Ph (to order): 800-274-7581
www.healthletter.tufts.edu

Experts at Tufts University review and rank websites that contain nutrition information through a Tufts sponsored website.
http://navigator.tufts.edu

The American Dietetic Association offers lists of registered dietitians as well as other nutrition information on their website.
American Dietetic Association
216 W. Jackson Boulevard
Chicago, IL 60606-6995
Ph: 800-366-1655
www.eatright.org

Three books with reliable current information:

The American Dietetic Association's Complete Food & Nutrition Guide. Roberta Larson Duyff (Minnetonka, MN: Chronimed, 1998).

Understanding Nutrition. 8th ed. Eleanor Noss Whitney and Sharon Rady Rolfes (Belmont, CA: Wadsworth, 1998).

Lifestyle Nutrition. James M. Rippe and Johanna T. Dwyer, eds. (Boston: Blackwell Scientific, 2000).

Exercise equipment
All Pro Exercise Products, Inc.
P.O. Box 8268
Longboat Key, FL 34228
Ph: 800-735-9287 or 941-387-9432
Fax: 941-387-7901
www.allproweights.com

Country Technology, Inc.
P.O. Box 87
Gays Mills, WI 54631
Ph: 608-735-4718
Fax: 608-735-4859

Fitness Distributors
25 Washington Street
Natick, MA 01760
Ph: 508-653-1882 or 800-244-1882
Fax: 508-650-0448

Intellbell's PowerBlock
1819 South Cedar Avenue
Owatonna, MN 55060
Ph: 800-446-5215
www.powerblock.com

Keiser Sports Health Equipment
2470 South Cherry Avenue
Fresno, CA 93706-9952
Ph: 559-256-8000 or 800-888-7009
Fax: 559-256-8100
www.keiser.com

MC Sports
3070 Shaffer Street, SE
Grand Rapids, MI 49512
Ph: 800-626-1762
Fax: 616-942-1973

Paragon Sports, Inc.
867 Broadway
New York, NY 10003
Ph: 212-255-8036
Fax: 212-929-1831

Exercise information

We believe that Bob Anderson's book on stretching, *Stretching 20th Anniversary: An Extensive Book on Stretching* (Bolinas, CA: Shelter Publications, August 2000), is the best book on stretching.

The National Strength and Conditioning Association lists certified personal trainers on their website.

National Strength and Conditioning Association
1955 N. Union Boulevard
Colorado Springs, CO 80909
Ph: 719-632-6722 or 800-805-6826
Fax: 719-632-6367
www.nsca.com

Osteoporosis

The National Osteoporosis Foundation (NOF)
1232 22nd Street, NW
Washington, DC 20037-1292
Ph: 202-223-2226 or 800-223-9944
www.nof.org

Complementary medicine

The following are two books on complementary medicine:

Ayurvedic Healing. David Frawley. (Salt Lake City, UT: Morson Publishing, 1991).

The Arthritis Foundation's Guide to Alternative Therapies. Judith Horstman. (Atlanta: Arthritis Foundation, 1999).

The following organizations can give you more information on a particular area of interest as well as help you find a qualified practitioner.

American Academy of Medical Acupuncture
4929 Wilshire Boulevard, Suite 428
Los Angeles, CA 90010
Ph: 323-937-5514
E-mail: JDOWDEN@prodigy.net
www.medicalacupuncture.org

American Association of Oriental Medicine (AAOM)
433 Front Street
Catasuagua, PA 18032
Ph: 888-500-7999 or 610-266-1433
www.aaom.org

The American Chiropractic Association
1701 Clarendon Boulevard
Arlington, VA 22209
Ph: 800-986-4636
www.amerchiro.org

American Occupational Therapy Association
4720 Montgomery Lane
P.O. Box 31220
Bethesda, MD 20824-1220
Ph: 301-652-2682 or TDD or 800-377-8555
Fax: 301-652-7711
www.aota.org

American Physical Therapy Association
1111 North Fairfax Street
Alexandria, VA 22314-1488
Ph: 703-684-APTA (2782) or 800-999-APTA
Fax: 703-684-7343
www.apta.org

The Ayurvedic Institute
11311 Menaul, NE
Albuquerque, NM 87112
Ph: 505-291-9698
www.ayurveda.com

The National Certification Commission for Acupuncture
and Oriental Medicine
11 Canal Center Plaza, Suite 300

Alexandria, VA 22314
Ph: 703-548-9004
www.nccaom.org

Regarding DMSO:
Stanley Jacob, M.D.
Gerlinger Professor, School of Medicine
Oregon Health Sciences University
3181 Sam Jackson Park Road, SW
Portland, OR 97201-3098

Yoga Journal
Yoga Teachers Directory and Source
2054 University Avenue
Berkeley, CA 94704
Ph: 510-841-9200
Fax: 510-644-3101
www.yogajournal.com

An excellent Tai Chi program for arthritis has been developed by Dr. Paul Lam, an Australian medical doctor and a Tai Chi Gold Medal winner who took up Tai Chi more than 20 years ago to reduce the impact of arthritis on his own life. It is supported by the Australian Arthritis Foundation. To learn more about Dr. Lam's program, check out www.taichiforarthritis.com on the Web. To purchase one of his videos, contact Tai Chi Productions.

Tai Chi Productions
P.O. Box 752
Butler, NJ 07405
Ph: 973-283-9698
Fax: 800-889-2082
www.taichiproductions.com

References

General arthritis

Coggon, D.; P. Croft; S. Kellingray; D. Barrett; M. McLaren; and C. Cooper. 2000. "Occupational physical activities and osteoarthritis of the knee." *Arthritis and Rheumatism* 43(7): 1443–49.

Ettinger, W. H., Jr.; and R. F. Afable. 1994. "Physical disability from knee osteoarthritis: the role of exercise as an intervention." *Medicine and Science in Sports and Exercise* 26(12): 1435–40.

Ettinger, W. H.; M. A. Davis; J. M. Neuhaus; and K. P. Mallon. 1994. "Long-term physical functioning in persons with knee osteoarthritis from NHANES I: effects of comorbid conditions." *Journal of Clinical Epidemiology* 47(7): 809–15.

Felson, D. T. 1995. "Weight and osteoarthritis." *Journal of Rheumatology* 22(suppl. 43): 7–9.

Felson, D. T.; and Y. Zhang. 1998. "An update on the epidemiology of knee and hip osteoarthritis with a view to prevention." *Arthritis and Rheumatism* 41(8): 1343–55.

Felson, D. T.; Y. Zhang; J. M. Anthony; A. Naimark; and J. Anderson. 1992. "Weight loss reduced the risk for symptomatic knee osteoarthritis in women." *Annals of Internal Medicine* 116: 535–39.

Felson, D. T.; Y. Zhang; M. T. Hannah; A. Naimark; B. Weissman; P. Aliabadi; and D. Levy. 1997. "Risk factors for incident radiographic knee osteoarthritis in the elderly." *Arthritis and Rheumatism* 40(4): 728–33.

Guidelines, American College of Rheumatology 2000. "Recommendations for the medical management of osteoarthritis of the hip and knee." *Arthritis and Rheumatism* 43(9): 1905–15.

Kerrigan, D. C.; M. K. Todd; and P. O. Riley. 1998. "Knee osteoarthritis and high-heeled shoes." *The Lancet* 351: 1399–1401.

Lawrence, R. C.; C. G. Helmick; F. C. Arnett; R. A. Deyo; D. T. Felson; E. H. Giannini; S. P. Heyse; R. Hirsch; M. C. Hochberg; G. G. Hunder; M. H. Liang; S. R. Pillemer; V. D. Steen; and F. Wolfe. 1998. "Estimates of the prevalence of arthritis and selected musculoskeletal disorders in the United States." *Arthritis and Rheumatism* 41(5): 778–99.

McAlindon, T. E.; C. Cooper; J. R. Kirwan; and P. A. Dieppe. 1993. "Determinants of disability in osteoarthritis of the knee." *Annals of the Rheumatic Diseases* 52: 258–62.

Oliveria, S. A.; D. T. Felson; P. A. Cirillo; J. I. Reed; and A. M. Walker. 1999. "Body weight, body mass index, and incident symptomatic osteoarthritis of the hand, hip, and knee." *Epidemiology* 10: 161–66.

Rejeski, W. J.; T. Craven; W. H. J. Ettinger; M. McFarlane; and S. Shumaker. 1996. "Self-efficacy and pain in disability with osteoarthritis of the knee." *Journal of Gerontology. Series B, Psychological Sciences and Social Sciences* 51B(1): 24–29.

Rejeski, W. J.; W. H. Ettinger; K. Martin; and T. Morgan. 1998. "Treating disability in knee osteoarthritis with exercise therapy: a central role for self-efficacy and pain." *Arthritis Care and Research* 11(2): 94–101.

Slemenda, C.; K. D. Brandt; D. K. Heilman; S. Mazzuca; E. M. Braunsttein; B. P. Katz; and F. D. Wolinsky. 1997. "Quadriceps weakness and osteoarthritis of the knee." *Annals of Internal Medicine* 127(2): 97–104.

Slemenda, C.; D. K. Heilman; K. D. Brandt; B. P. Katz; S. Mazzuca; E. M. Braunsttein; and D. Byrd. 1998. "Reduced quadriceps strength relative to body weight." *Arthritis and Rheumatism* 41(11): 1951–59.

Van Baar, M. E.; J. Dekker; A. M. Lemmens; R. A. B. Oostendorp; and W. J. J. Bijlsma. 1998. "Pain and disability in patients with osteoarthritis of hip or knee: the relationship with articular, kinesiological, and psychological characteristics." *Journal of Rheumatology* 25: 125–33.

Nutrition

Belch, J.; and A. Hill. 2000. "Evening primrose oil and borage oil in rheumatologic conditions." *American Journal of Clinical Nutrition* 71 (suppl.): 352S–356S.

Cleland, L. G.; C. L. Hill; and M. J. James. 1995. "Diet and arthritis." *Bailliere's Clinical Rheumatology* 9(4): 771–85.

Connor, W. E. 2000. "Importance of n-3 fatty acids in health and disease." *American Journal of Clinical Nutrition* 71(suppl.): 171S–175S.

Edmonds, S. E.; P. G. Winyard; R. Guo; B. Kidd; P. Merry; A. Langrish-Smith; C. Hansen; S. Ramm; and D. R. Blake. 1997. "Putative analgesic activity of repeated oral doses of vitamin E in the treatment of rheumatoid arthritis. Results of a prospective placebo controlled double blind trial." *Annals of the Rheumatic Diseases* 56: 649–55.

Felson, D. T.; and T. E. McAlindon. 2000. "Glucosamine and chondroitin for osteoarthritis: to recommend or not to recommend?" *Arthritis Care and Research* 13(4): 179–82.

Hansen, G. V. O.; L. Nielsen; E. Kluger; M. Thysen; H Emmertsen; K. Stengaard-Pedersen; W. L. Hansen; B. Unger; and P. W. Andersen. 1996. "Nutritional status of Danish rheumatoid arthritis patients and effects of a diet adjusted in energy intake, fish-meal and antioxidants." *Sandinavian Journal of Rheumatology* 25: 325–30.

Heliovaara, M.; P. Knekt; K. Aho; R. K. Aaran; G. Alfthan; and W. Aromaa. 1994. "Serum antioxidants and the risk of rheumatoid arthritis." *Annals of the Rheumatic Diseases* 53(1): 51–53.

Henderson, C. J.; and R. S. Panush. 1999. "Diets, dietary supplements, and nutritional therapies in rheumatic diseases." *Rheumatic Disease Clinics of North America* 25(4): 937–68.

Huang, M.; C. Chen; T. Chen; and M. Weng. 2000. "The effects of weight reduction on the rehabilitation of patients with knee osteoarthritis and obesity." *Arthritis Care and Research* 13(6): 398–405.

James, M. J.; and L. G. Cleland (1997). "Dietary n-3 fatty acids and therapy for rheumatoid arthritis." *Seminars in Arthritis and Rheumatism* 27: 85–97.

James, M. J.; R. A. Gibson; and L. G. Cleland. 2000. "Dietary polyunsaturated fatty acids and inflammatory mediator production." *American Journal of Clinical Nutrition* 71(suppl.): 343S–348S.

Kjeldsen-Kragh, J.; M. Haugen; C. F. Borchgrevink; E. Laerum; M. Eek; P. Mowinkel; K. Hovi; and O. Forre. 1991. "Controlled trial of fasting and one-year vegetarian diet in rheumatoid arthritis." *The Lancet* 338: 899–902.

Kowasari, B.; S. K. Finnie; R. L. Carter; J. Love; P. Katz; S. Longley; and R. S. Panush. 1983. "Assessment of the diet of patients with rheumatoid arthritis and osteoarthritis." *Journal of the American Dietetic Association* 82(6): 657–59.

Kremer, J. M. 2000. "n-3 fatty acid supplements in rheumatoid arthritis." *American Journal of Clinical Nutiriton* 71(suppl.): 349S–351S.

Kremer, J. M.; D. A. Lawrence; W. Jubiz; R. DiGiacomo; R. Rynes; L. E. Bartholomew; and M. Sherman. 1990. "Dietary fish oil and olive oil supplementation in patients with rheumatoid arthritis. Clinical and immunologic effects." *Arthritis and Rheumatism* 33(6): 810–20.

Kremer, J. M.; D. A. Lawrence; G. F. Petrillo; L. Litts; P. M. Mullaly; R. I. Rynes; R. P. Stocker; N. Parhami; N. S. Greenstein; B. R. Fuchs; A. Mathur; D. R. Robinson; R. I. Sperling; and J. Bigaouette. 1995. "Effects on high-dose fish oil on rheumatoid arthritis after stopping nonsteroidal anti-inflammatory drugs." *Arthritis and Rheumatism* 8: 1107–14.

Kris-Etherton, P. M.; D. S. Taylor; S. Yu-Poth; P. Huth; K. Moriarty; V. Fishell; and R. L. Hargrove. 2000. "Polyunsaturated fatty acids in the food chain in the United States." *American Journal of Clinical Nutrition* 71(suppl.): 179S–188S.

Lau, C. S.; K. D. Morley; and J. J. F. Belch. 1993. "Effects of fish oil supplementation on nonsteroidal anti-inflammatory drug requirement in patients with mild rheumatoid arhtritis—a double-blind placebo controlled study." *British Journal of Rheumatology* 32: 982–89.

Leventhal, L. J.; E. G. Boyce; and R. B. Zurier. 1993. "Treatment of rheumatoid arthritis with black currant seed oil." *British Journal of Rheumatology* 33: 847–52.

Levanthal, L. J.; E. G. Boyce; and R. B. Zurier. 1993. "Treatment of rheumatoid arthritis with gammalinolenic acid." *Annals of Internal Medicine* 119(9): 867–73.

Linos, A.; V. G. Kaklamani; E. Kaklamani; Y. Koumantaki; E. Giziaki; S. Papazoglou; and C. S. Mantzoros. 2000. "Dietary factors in relation to rheumatoid arthritis: a role for olive oil and cooked vegetables?" *American Journal of Clinical Nutrition* 70(6): 1077–82.

McAlindon, T.; and D. T. Felson. 1997. "Nutrition: risk factors for osteo-arthritis." *Annals of the Rheumatic Diseases* 56(7): 397–400.

McAlindon, T.; M. P. LaValley; J. P. Gulin; and D. T. Felson. 2000. "Glu-cosamine and chondroitin for treatment of osteoarthritis: a systematic quality assessment and meta-analysis." *Journal of the American Medical Association* 283: 1469–75.

McAlindon, T. E.; D. T. Felson; Y. Zhang; M. T. Hannan; P. Aliabadi; B. Weiss-man; D. Rush; and P. Wilson. 1996. "Relation of dietary intake and serum levels of vitamin D to progression of osteoarthritis of the knee among participants in the Framingham study." *Annals of Internal Medicine* 125: 353–59.

McAlindon, T. E.; P. Jacques; Y. Zhang; M. T. Hannan; P. Aliabadi; B. Weiss-man; et al. 1996. "Do antioxidant micronutrients protect against the devel-opment and progression of knee osteoarthritis?" *Arthritis and Rheumatism* 39: 648–56.

Panush, R. S.; R. L. Carter; P. Katz; B. Kowsari; S. Longley; and S. Finnie. 1983. "Diet therapy for rheumatoid arthritis." *Arthritis and Rheumatism* 26(4): 462–71.

Shapiro, J. A.; T. D. Koepsell; L. F. Voigt; C. E. Dugowson; M. Kestin; and J. L. Nelson. 1996. "Diet and rheumatoid arthritis in women: a possible protective effect of fish consumption." *Epidemiology* 7: 256–63.

Skoldstam, L.; O. Borjesson; A. Kjallman; B. Seiving; and B. Akesson. 1992. "Effect of six months of fish oil supplementation in stable rheumatoid arthritis: a double-blind, controlled study." *Scandinavian Journal of Rheuma-tology* 21: 178–85.

Volker, D.; P. Fitzgerald; G. Major; and M. Garg. 2000. "Efficacy of fish oil concentrate in the treatment of rheumatoid arthritis." *Journal of Rheuma-tology* 27: 2343–46.

Exercise

Baker, K.; and T. McAlindon. 2000. "Exercise for knee osteoarthritis." *Current Opinion in Rheumatology* 12: 456–63.

Baker, K.; M. Nelson; D. Felson; J. Layne; R. Sarno; and R. Roubenoff. 2001. "The efficacy of home-based, progressive strength training in older adults with knee osteoarthritis." *Journal of Rheumatology* 28: 1655–65.

Deyle, G. D.; N. E. Henderson; R. L. Matekel; M. G. Ryder; M. B. Garber; and S. C. Allison. 2000. "Effectiveness of manual physical therapy and exercise in osteoarthritis of the knee: a randomized controlled trial." *Annals of Internal Medicine* 132(3): 173–81.

Ettinger, W. H., Jr.; R. Burns; S. P. Messier; W. Applegate; W. J. Rejeski; T. Morgan; S. Shumaker; M. J. Berry; M. O'Toole; J. Monu; and T. Craven. 1997. "A randomized trial comparing aerobic exercise and resistance exercise with a health education program in older adults with knee osteoarthritis." *Journal of the American Medical Association* 277(1): 25–31.

Hakkinen, A.; T. Sokka; A. Kotaniemi; and P. Hannonen. 2001. "A randomized two-year study of the effects of dynamic strength training on muscle strength, disease activity, functional capacity, and bone mineral density in early rheumatoid arthritis." *Arthritis and Rheumatism* 44(3): 515–22.

Kovar, P. A.; J. P. Allegrante; R. MacKenzie; M. G. E. Peterson; B. Gutin; and M. E. Charlson. 1992. "Supervised fitness walking in patients with osteoarthritis of the knee." *Annals of Internal Medicine* 116(7): 529–34.

Messier, S. P.; R. F. Looser; M. N. Mitchell; G. Valle; T. P. Morgan; W. J. Rejeski; and W. H. Ettinger. 2000. "Exercise and weight loss in obese older adults with knee osteoarthritis: a preliminary study." *Journal of the American Geriatric Society* 48: 1062–72.

Minor, M. A.; J. E. Hewett; R. R. Webel; S. K. Anderson; and D. R. Kay. 1989. "Efficacy of physical conditioning exercise in patients with rheumatoid arthritis and osteoarthritis." *Arthritis and Rheumatism* 32(11): 1396–1405.

O'Reilly, S. C.; A. Jones; K. R. Muir; and M. Doherty. 1998. "Quadriceps weakness in knee osteoarthritis: the effect on pain and disability." *Annals of Rheumatic Diseases* 57: 588–94.

O'Reilly, S. C.; K. R. Muir; and M. Doherty. 1999. "Effectiveness of home exercise on pain and disability from osteoarthritis of the knee: a randomized controlled trial." *Annals of the Rheumatic Diseases* 58: 15–19.

Rall, L. C.; S. N. Meydani; J. J. Kehayias; B. Dawson-Hughes; and R. Roubenoff. 1996. "The effect of progressive resistance training in rheumatoid arthritis." *Arthritis and Rheumatism* 39: 415–26.

Rall, L. C.; C. J. Rosen; G. Dolnikowski; W. J. Hartman; N. Lungren; L. W. Abad; C. A. Dinarello; and R. Roubenoff. "Protein metabolism in rheumatoid arthritis and aging: effects of muscle strength training and tumor necrosis factor-alpha." *Arthritis and Rheumatism* 39: 1115–24.

Rejeski, W. J.; W. H. Ettinger; K. Martin; and T. Morgan. 1998. "Treating disability in knee osteoarthritis with exercise therapy: a central role for self-efficacy and pain." *Arthritis Care and Research* 11(2): 94–101.

van Baar, M. E.; W. J. J. Assendelft; J. Dekker; R. A. B. Oostendorp; and J. W. J. Bijlsma. 1999. "Effectiveness of exercise therapy in patients with osteoarthritis of the hip or knee a systematic review of randomized clinical trials." *Arthritis and Rheumatism* 43(7): 1361–69.

van Baar, M. E.; J. Dekker; R. A. B. Oostendorp; D. Bijl; T. B. Voorn; J. A. M. Lemmens; and J. W. J. Bijlsma. 1998. "The effectiveness of exercise therapy in patients with osteoarthritis of the hip or knee: a randomized clinical trial." *Journal of Rheumatology* 25: 2432–39.

Complementary therapy

Berman, B. M.; J. P. Swyers; and J. Ezzo. 2000. "The evidence for acupuncture as a treatment for rheumatologic conditions." *Rheumatic Disease Clinics of North America* 26(1): 103–15.

Garfinkel, M.; and H. R. Schumacher. 2000. "Yoga." *Rheumatic Disease Clinics of North America* 26(1): 125–32.

Garfinkel, M. S.; H. R. Schumacher; A. Husain; M. Levy; and R. A. Reshetar. 1994. "Evaluation of a yoga based regimen for treatment of osteoarthritis of the hands." *Journal of Rheumatology* 21: 2341–43.

Hartman, C. A.; T. M. Manos; C. Winter; D. M. Hartman; L. Baiqing; and J. C. Smith. 2000. "Effects of T'ai Chi training on function and quality of life indicators in older adults with osteoarthritis." *Journal of the American Geriatric Society* 48: 1553–59.

Lan, C.; J. Lai; S. Chen; and M. Wong. 1998. "12-month Tai Chi training in the elderly: its effect on health fitness." *Medicine and Science in Sports and Exercise* 30(3): 345–51.

Lan, C.; J. Lai; S. Chen; and M. Wong. 2000. "Tai Chi Chuan to improve muscular strength and endurance in elderly individuals: a pilot study." *Archives of Physical Medicine and Rehabilitation* 81(5): 604–7.

Ramos-Remus, C.; C. A. Watters; L. Dyke; M. E. Suarez-Alamazor; and A. S. Russell. 1999. "Assessment of health locus of control in the use of nonconventional remedies by patients with rheumatic diseases." *Journal of Rheumatology* 26(11): 2468–74.

Wolf, S. L.; H. X. Barnhart; N. G. Kutnear; E. McNeely; C. Coogler; T. Xu; and A. F. Group. 1996. "Reducing frailty and falls in older persons: an investigation of Tai Chi and computerized balance training." *Journal of the American Geriatric Society* 4: 489–97.

Wolfson, L.; R. Whipple; C. Derby; J. Judge; M. King; P. Amerman; J. Schmidt; and D. Smyers. 1996. "Balance and strength training in older adults: intervention gains and Tai Chi maintenance." *Journal of the American Geriatric Society* 44: 498–506.

Surgery

Dieppe, P.; H.-D. Basler; J. Chard; P. Croft; J. Dixon; M. Hurley; S. Lohmander; and H. Raspe. 1999. "Knee replacement surgery for osteoarthritis: effectiveness, practice variations, indications and possible determinants of utilization." *Rheumatology* 38: 73–83.

Fortin, P. R.; A. E. Clarke; L. Joseph; M. H. Liang; M. Tanzer; D. Ferland; C. Phillips; A. J. Partridge; P. Belisle; A. H. Fossel; N. Mahomed; C. B. Sledge; and K. J. N. Katz. 1999. "Outcomes of total hip and knee replacement." *Arthritis and Rheumatism* 42(8): 1722–28.

Hawker, G.; J. Wright; P. Coyte; J. Paul; R. Dittus; R. Croxford; C. Bombardier; D. Heck; and D. Freund. 1998. "Health-related quality of life after knee replacement." *Journal of Bone and Joint Surgery.* British Volume 80-A(2): 163–73.

Shields, R. K.; L. J. Enloe; and K. C. Leo. 1999. "Health-related quality of life in patients with total hip or knee replacement." *Archives of Physical Medicine and Rehabilitation* 80: 572–79.

Walsh, M.; L. J. Woodhouse; S. G. Thomas; and E. Finch. 1998. "Physical impairment and functional limitations: a comparison of individuals 1 year after total knee arthroplasty with control subjects." *Physical Therapy* 78(3): 248–58.

Index

■

Miriam E. Nelson, Ph.D., is the author of the international best-sellers *Strong Women Stay Young; Strong Women Stay Slim; Strong Women, Strong Bones;* and *Strong Women Eat Well.* She is Associate Professor of Nutrition at the Friedman School of Nutrition Science and Policy and director of the Center for Physical Activity and Nutrition at Tufts University. Dr. Nelson is a Fellow of the American College of Sports Medicine, an honor reserved for those who have demonstrated superior leadership and research in the field of exercise. Her original research papers on nutrition and exercise have been published in distinguished peer-reviewed journals, including the *Journal of the American Medical Association.* In 1994 she was named a Brookdale National Fellow, a prestigious award given annually to only five or six young scholars in the field of aging. She was a Bunting Fellow at Radcliffe College in 1997–1998. In 2000, *Strong Women, Strong Bones* received the Books for a Better Life Award from the Multiple Sclerosis Society for best wellness book. Dr. Nelson has been featured on many television and radio shows including *The Oprah Winfrey Show, The Today Show, Good Morning America,* CNN, and *Fresh Air.* She is the founder of www.StrongWomen.com. She lives in Concord, Massachusetts, with her husband and three children.

Kristin R. Baker, Ph.D., is a Doctoral Fellow at the National Institutes of Health Multipurpose Arthritis and Musculoskeletal Diseases Center at the Boston University Medical School. She received her doctorate from the School of Nutrition Science and Policy at Tufts University under the guidance of Drs. Ronenn Roubenoff and Miriam Nelson. Her doctoral thesis was an investigation of the effects of strength training on knee osteoarthritis. Dr. Baker received research awards from the Arthritis Foundation, Life Fitness Academy, and the American Federation of Aging /Glenn Foundation to conduct this research. She currently conducts research on complementary treatments for arthritis, and lives in Concord, Massachusetts with her husband and daughter.

Ronenn Roubenoff, M.D., M.H.S., trained in internal medicine, rheumatology, and clinical epidemiology at Johns Hopkins University. He then continued his education in nutrition at Tufts University and currently focuses his research on the interactions of nutrition, exercise, and hormonal and immune regulators of metabolism in chronic disease and aging. He is currently Chief of the Nutrition, Exercise Physiology, and Sarcopenia Laboratory at the Jean Mayer USDA Human Nutrition Research Center on Aging at Tufts University and is Associate Professor of Medicine and Nutrition at Tufts. Dr. Roubenoff is an author of more than one hundred scientific papers and the recipient of many awards, including the American College of Rheumatology Senior Scholar Award, the Pew Foundation National Nutrition Scholar, and the Tufts University Distinguished Faculty Award. He is also a member of the medical honor societies Alpha Omega Alpha and Delta Omega. He practices rheumatology and nutrition at the Itzhak Perlman Family Arthritis Center at New England Medical Center in Boston, where his patients have recognized him with the Oliver Smith Award for Extraordinary Service and Caring over a dozen times. Dr. Roubenoff lives in Sharon, Massachusetts, with his wife, son, dog, and two cats.

Lawrence Lindner, M.A., is the executive editor of the *Tufts University Health & Nutrition Letter.* He also penned the "Eating Right" column for *The Washington Post* for three years and currently freelances for a variety of magazines on health, travel, and other subjects. He lives in Hingham, Massachusetts, with his wife and son.